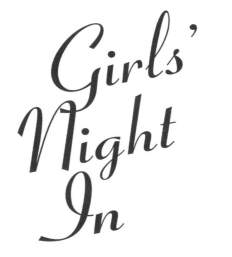

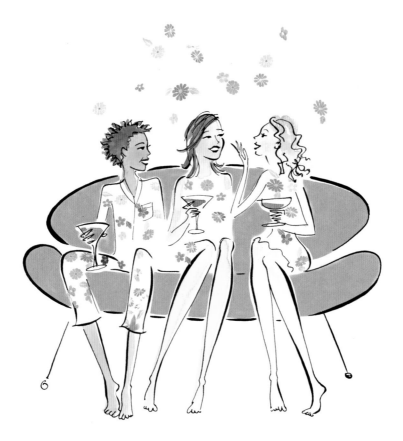

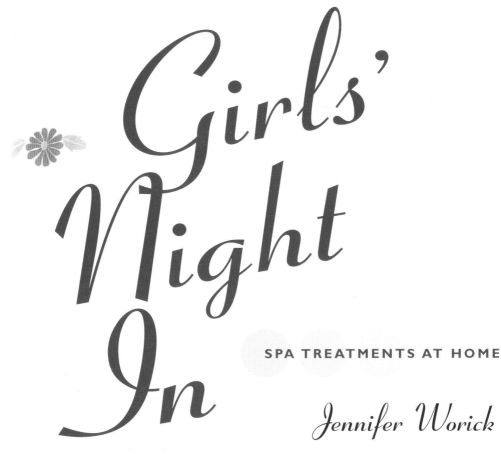

Girls' Night In

SPA TREATMENTS AT HOME

Jennifer Worick

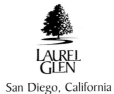

LAUREL GLEN

San Diego, California

Laurel Glen Publishing
An imprint of the Advantage Publishers Group
5880 Oberlin Drive, San Diego, CA 92121-4794
www.laurelglenbooks.com

Produced by PRC Publishing Limited,
The Chrysalis Building,
Bramley Road, London W10 6SP, U.K.
An imprint of **Chrysalis** Books Group

All notations of errors or omissions should be addressed to Laurel Glen Publishing,
Editorial Department, at the above address. All other correspondence (author inquiries,
permissions, and rights) concerning the content of this book should be addressed to
PRC Publishing Limited, The Chrysalis Building, Bramley Road, London W10 6SP,
United Kingdom. A member of the Chrysalis Group plc.

Library of Congress Cataloging-in-Publication Data

Worick, Jennifer.
 Girl's night in : spa treatments at home / Jennifer Worick
  p. cm.
Includes index.
ISBN 1-59223-276-0
1. Beauty, Personal. 2. Cosmetics. 3. Women-Health and hygiene. I. Title.
RA778.W83 2004
646.7'042-dc22
                        2004053206

Printed and bound in Malaysia

1 2 3 4 5 08 07 06 05 04

All illustrations © Chrysalis Image Library / Robyn Neild.

Contents

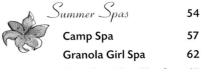

Introduction

If you're reading this, you probably already know the sublime pleasures to be found at a spa—or at least in a facial treatment at home. Or even by washing your face after a particularly crazy night of barhopping.

Regardless of your level of "spa-aptitude," gals love to be pampered. Sometimes you have to treat yourself, sometimes you have to do it on a budget, and sometimes you have to take a friend by the hand and force her to indulge herself.

Girls' Night In is a way to accomplish all three. The best party I've thrown in recent memory was a spa party I hosted on Super Bowl Sunday, where I invited eight of my best girlfriends.

I created a "Menu of Services" on the computer, listing all the treatments that would be available (i.e., that I could do reasonably well without injury). These included a paraffin hand dip followed by a manicure, a spa pedicure complete with reflexology massage, customized facials, and glycolic facial peels (one of my friends, a dermatologist, brought the necessary tools).

Then there was the food. I layered yogurt, fruit, and granola and created a delicious parfait for a great alternative to the usual Super Bowl snacks (see page 63). We had juice and water infused with lemon and strawberries. As the day went on, we switched to cosmopolitans (see page 88) and homemade sushi rolls. We adjourned, buffed and polished, to my living room, where we proceeded to get ripped and watch episodes of *Sex and the City* on DVD. We paused to check in on the halftime show. Could the day be any more glorious?

Well, yes. I sent the ladies home with goody bags filled with cuticle cream, shower caps, and a wacky shade of nail polish. It sounds extravagant, but I had much of the necessary ingredients on hand. If you happen to have a bin of nail polish, various face masks that you've sampled but don't work with your particular skin type, and mellow spa tunes (although I draw the line at Enya and sounds of water lapping against rocks), you have the stuff for a spectacular day of luxurious indulgences.

You don't need to go to a fancy-schmancy day spa to have a little quality girl bonding. Host your own party. There's obvious benefits. Juicy gossip won't be overheard by nosy society mavens. You don't have to leave your house, and consequently, you don't have to change out of your pajamas. And you know that everything you are making is fresh and customized for you and your friends.

The Basics of Skin Care

The lesson here? You must take care of your skin! I had a friend who revealed to me that she never washed her face. Ever. I am still recovering from the shock of that admission. Seriously. How can a woman who's almost thirty go without washing her face, even if she doesn't wear makeup or sweat at the gym? She explained it by saying that she's always had good skin and that the steam of the shower cleansed her face sufficiently. Um, what? You may indeed have always had good skin with a minimum of effort, but your skin changes as you age. It may become drier or acne-prone or just show signs of aging. You can reduce fine lines and improve your skin's overall texture by a simple daily regimen accompanied by a weekly face mask or exfoliant.

That's where I come in.

If you are a newbie when it comes to all this extreme self-care, allow me to break it down for you. I think there are three basic parts to good skin care.

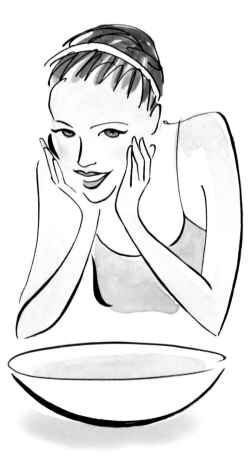

CLEANSING: Cleansers have come a long way! Bar soap or cold cream can suffice, but there are a lot of great options on the market now for all skin types. If your skin is dry, go for a creamier cleanser with minimal foaming action. If you are a bit on the oily side, you can indulge in a cleanser that's soapier (with lots of bubbling action) or has a bit of scrub to it. Regardless of what you use, rub it in thoroughly (but gently) to remove dirt and makeup and then rinse thoroughly with water to remove all traces of the cleanser. Do not wash your face with hot water, which can be extremely drying to the skin. Stick to warm water only.

TONING: This isn't always considered essential, but I like it. It can remove any residue from the cleansing step, close the pores, soothe the skin, restore the pH balance, and prep it for moisturizer. If you have dry skin, shy away from toners containing alcohol. Look instead for gentle ingredients like witch hazel. Oilier skin may benefit from the bracing effect of an alcohol-based toner. Use a cotton ball or pad to swipe toner over your face, paying particular attention to your T-zone (the oilier area on the forehead and middle of the face).

MOISTURIZING: All skin types should be moisturized daily! Good moisturizers do not clog pores. If you have dry skin, you can go for a creamier formulation, and oilier skins would do better with a lighter lotion or gel moisturizer. Don't be shy. Ask for free samples when deciding between products. Companies and stores want repeat customers who are happy with their products, not someone who returns a partially used jar of a pricey confection.

SUNSCREEN: Applying sunscreen on a daily basis is also critical. For whatever reason, I do not like to wear moisturizer to bed if it contains sunscreen. I'd rather have some other secret weapon that will be repairing the skin, treating fine lines, or washing my dishes. Okay, a girl can dream about the latter. Anyway, many moisturizers contain sunscreen, so you can combine these two steps. I love them. You can also opt to smear on a thin layer of sunscreen in addition to your moisturizer. Even if you are wearing a hat or staying inside or it's overcast, wear your sunscreen! Make it a habit and you will enjoy many years of creamy skin that looks ten years younger than it is. I swear. My skin is my most admired feature. I am in my mid-thirties and am constantly mistaken for someone in her late twenties. It's all about the sunscreen and, obviously, my youthful attitude to life.

MASKS: Masks exist to address every skin type or skin issue. Whether you have dry, oily, sun-damaged, blemish-prone, or uneven skin, different masks can be formulated (even at home) to treat your skin on a weekly basis or as needed.

EXFOLIANTS: Your skin might be dull or flaky not because you need a heavier moisturizer, but because you need to slough off dead skin cells.

Using an exfoliant regularly will ensure that you are keeping your skin in great condition. My favorite products can be used in the shower. I just rub a little all over my face and leave it on for several minutes. I like "natural" ones that contain ground-up kernels, seeds, or shells and contain fruit enzymes that exfoliate without much abrasion to the skin.

Don't wait for someone else to pamper you; do it yourself and do it a heck of a lot cheaper than any fancy spa in an exotic locale.

A Dictionary for the Spa-Challenged

Here are just a few terms you might come across, should you embrace the spa life. It's rather subjective and limited, as there are scientific and alternative treatments and techniques being introduced in spas all the time. I just want you to get your feet wet so that the next time you visit a spa, you'll be able to navigate the most extensive of treatment menus with ease!

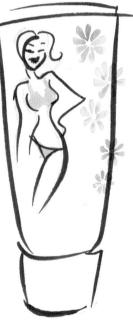

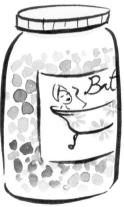

ACUPRESSURE: An alternative therapy that uses manual pressure to relieve pain and promote health.

ACUPUNCTURE: A form of Chinese alternative medicine that treats disorders by inserting needles into the skin at points where the flow of energy is thought to be blocked, helping to release it.

AESTHETICIAN: A certified spa professional who specializes in skin care.

ALEXANDER TECHNIQUE: A method of improving posture that involves developing awareness of it.

AROMATHERAPY: The use of essential oils to soothe the mind and body. Oils are often used in massages, but can be helpful when used alone or in a bath.

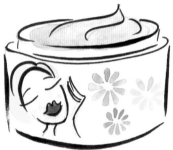

AYURVEDA: A 5,000-year-old system of healing that originated in India. The five elements (space, air, fire, water, and earth) manifest themselves in three doshas: Vata (space and air), Pitta (fire and water), and Kapha (water and earth). See page 71 for more information.

BRAZILIAN: The mother of all bikini waxes, this one removes all hair south of your border. Ouch. Make sure you want to commit to this because once the wax is on, there's no going back.

CARRIER OIL: A high-quality oil like olive oil or sweet almond oil. A few drops of essential oil can be put into a few tablespoons or an ounce of carrier oil to dilute the powerful essential oil.

CHAKRA: One of seven major energy centers situated from the base of the spine to the crown of the head, plus scores of minor centers throughout the body. These correspond to nerve clusters where nerves from every part of the body join the spinal cord (see page 69).

COLOR THERAPY: At its most basic, color therapy uses color, which affects our moods and emotions, to address any imbalances in the body's energy patterns that might lead to poor emotional or physical health. See page 89 for more information.

CRYSTAL THERAPY: Crystal therapy falls under the category of vibrational medicine. Crystals embody light, water, and minerals and act as a sort of lens to channel color and energy into the body. Different crystals are used to address different ailments.

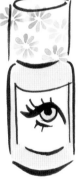

ESSENTIAL OIL: This is a very powerful form of a plant, herb, or flower. Using different essential oils in lotions, water, and carrier oils can make you feel better. When handling essential oils, keep the pure essential oils away from your skin. They are very powerful by themselves. Mix them with something else before applying them to your skin.

EXFOLIATE: The body sheds skin cells constantly. Using a body or face scrub can help your body exfoliate, or remove, dead skin. Your skin will glow afterward.

FACIAL: A treatment to improve the skin on your face by deep-cleaning and moisturizing it. The usual procedure for a spa facial includes cleansing, steaming, extracting (actually removing blackheads and whiteheads), applying a mask, and moisturizing. A light massage is sometimes included in the steaming or moisturizing portion of the facial. I've included recipes for cleansers, masks, massage, and facial steams, so let yourself go crazy and do full-on facials for your friends during any spa night.

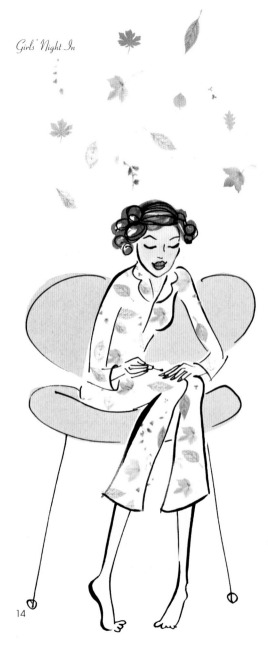

HYDROTHERAPY: The use of water for healing in spa treatment. Hydrotherapy has been used for centuries all over the world (think Roman baths and Japanese bathhouses) to treat all sorts of ailments. While it's much more scientific and high-tech in a spa, just taking a hot bath or shower will relieve stress; following it with a short, cold shower will stimulate you and perk you up. Many modern spa water effusions—low-pressure sprays of water—are based on the work of Father Sebastian Kneipp, a nineteenth-century Bavarian monk.

MANICURE: A manicure is a treatment for your hands and fingernails. It can include massage, pushing back or trimming cuticles, and shaping and polishing the nails. A French manicure includes whitening the tip and painting over the nail with a clear or lightly tinted polish. Acrylic nails are painted onto your own nails. When the acrylic hardens, the nails are buffed and shaped. Take care, however, as acrylic nails can weaken your natural fingernails.

MASK: A treatment for the face that addresses a particular skin-care problem. Masks can soothe, cleanse, exfoliate, reduce fine lines, moisturize, and treat acne or redness in the skin.

MASSAGE: This is a relaxing treatment that involves rubbing or kneading muscles. It is usually performed on the back, but any part of your body can be massaged. There are many types of massage treatments:

❀ *Aromatherapy:* This heavenly massage combines therapeutic aromatic essential oils with massage techniques (often Swedish).

❀ *Cranial-Sacral:* A massage that stimulates and manipulates the bones of the cranium. While you may not even feel the pressure, the massage improves the rhythmic flow of cerebrospinal fluid and is believed to treat a variety of physical ailments.

❀ *Hot Stone:* Heat from hot river stones penetrates your muscles as a massage therapist uses the rocks to work into tight muscles with long Swedish strokes.

❀ *Maya Abdominal:* Developed by Dr. Rosita Arvigo, this massage focuses on the position of the uterus and tonicity of uterine support.

❀ *Myofascial:* Also known as trigger point therapy, myofascial (from the Latin *myo,* "muscle," and *fascia,* "connective tissue") massages focus on applying pressure to tender muscle tissue to treat chronic pain in other areas of the body.

❀ *Reflexology:* A form of massage in which pressure is applied to certain parts of the feet and hands in order to promote relaxation and health elsewhere in the body.

❀ *Shiatsu:* A combination of pressure and assisted-stretching techniques, shiatsu does the body good. It can improve circulation, help with lymphatic drainage, and release toxins and tension in the muscles. Ahh.

❀ *Swedish:* A vigorous massage that features long and rolling strokes with gentle to firm pressure. Like shiatsu, Swedish massage can improve circulation and lymphatic fluid flow by helping to rid the body of toxins. And it's usually a full-body massage. What's not to like?

MEDICINE WHEEL: Basically, a medicine wheel resembles a crude wagon wheel. It is a circle with a cross inside it that can represent many things, including the four directions (north, south, east, west) and the four elements (water, earth, air, fire). The circle is a sacred shape in many cultures and is a symbol for the planets, the sun, the moon, the cycles of life, the seasons, the rotation of the earth, and the passage from day to night.

MENDHI: Popularized by Gwen Stefani and Madonna a few years back, these henna tattoos are still a fun and very attractive way to embellish your skin. An Indian tradition dating as far back as the twelfth century, this temporary stain is applied to the hands or feet, usually in ornate swirls and designs. It can last up to two weeks or more, but does eventually disappear altogether from the skin.

MOISTURIZER: A cream or lotion that hydrates and protects the skin.

PEDICURE: Like a manicure, a pedicure is a treat for your feet and toes. It usually includes a foot scrub, a massage, pushing back cuticles, and painting your toenails.

REIKI: A treatment in alternative medicine in which healing energy is channeled from the practitioner to the patient to enhance energy and reduce stress, pain, and fatigue.

STEAM: Steam is an excellent way to open your pores. Gyms and spas have steam rooms to open all the pores on your body. Put a towel over your head and lean over a sink full of hot water to open the pores on your face.

THALASSOTHERAPY: The use of seaweed in body treatments to draw out toxins.

THASSOTHERAPY: Not to be confused with thalassotherapy, it is the use of sea air or seawater in treating the body, mind, and spirit. Basically, all those Jane Austen characters from the Regency period who visited Brighton to "take the waters" were indulging in thassotherapy.

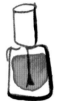

TONER: A light liquid that removes all traces of dirt or cleanser on the face. It also closes the pores and prepares the face for a moisturizer.

T-ZONE: The skin on your forehead and nose, which tends to be the oiliest area of the face.

YOGA: A system of breathing exercises and postures that promotes flexibility, stress reduction, and general wellness. Its benefits are many and its popularity continues to spread.

The Pantry

You may think that a pantry should only be used for storing food. There are a few other things you may want to keep on hand for various spa parties or when you just want to whip up an individual treat for yourself.

CARRIER OIL: Any high-quality vegetable oil such as almond, olive, wheat germ, grapeseed, or sesame. Carrier oils are the most effective way to dilute essential oils, and should be stored away from heat and light to ensure their freshness. Make blends in small amounts and use within a few months. They can be stored in the refrigerator for extended shelf life.

DISTILLED WATER: Not just for bomb shelters anymore! You can usually find this purified water next to the seltzer and other bottled waters at any supermarket. It's great for face spritzers, facial steams, and scented linen waters.

17

DRIED LAVENDER: You can find bags or jars of this at craft stores and gourmet grocery stores. It can be used in baths, dream pillows, facial steams, sachets, or even potpourri to evoke a farmhouse in Provence.

ESSENTIAL OILS: Keep your favorites on hand to enhance various products and change your mood. Lavender, lemon, and peppermint oils smell good. You can find them in your local health food store, beauty store, or drugstore. See page 20 for more information on the therapeutic properties of many essential oils.

FRUITS AND VEGETABLES: Bananas, papaya, cucumber, and avocado can be eaten or used in products for your skin. I love stuff that does double duty!

GLASS OR STAINLESS-STEEL BOWLS IN DIFFERENT SIZES: Make sure to start out with clean, dry bowls and utensils when mixing your potions.

HONEY: An excellent moisturizer (and it's tasty too).

LOTION: Look for unscented varieties you can doctor up. Leave a small vial of lotion next to every sink in your home and always moisturize after washing your hands. If you don't wash your hands, you have bigger things to worry about than dry skin.

MEASURING SPOONS AND CUPS: Measuring spoons and cups are necessary for mixing up your potions; those made of stainless steel and glass are preferable.

OATMEAL: A terrific natural exfoliant. Mix with honey for a quick face mask.

SEA SALT OR KOSHER SALT: Bigger than normal table salt, you can find this kind of salt at supermarkets, health food stores, gourmet food stores, and even some craft stores.

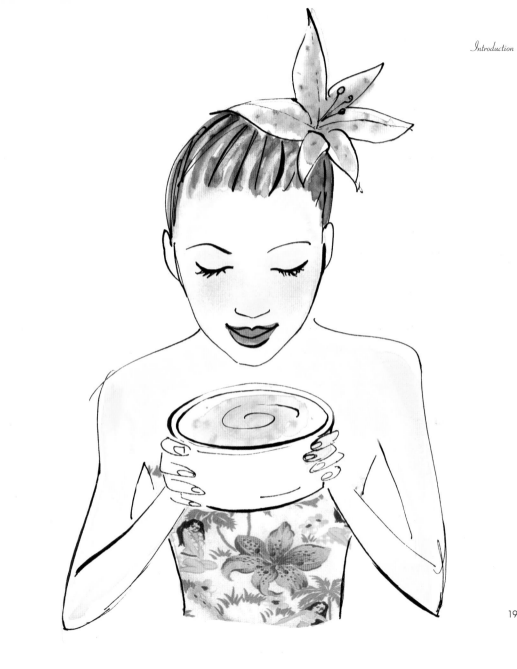

Essential Oils: More than Just a Pretty Smell

There are a whole lot more than the following oils, but these are my favorites, except for patchouli, which I hate but had to include because of its immense popularity among the hippie crowd. I use many of them in the concoctions in this book. Some oils have many uses, but in the interest of this book, I'm only listing the properties that relate to mood, skin, or hair. So while basil, bergamot, and verbena essential oils can be great insect repellents, I'm not mentioning that below. If you're interested in finding out more about essential oils, see the Resources section on page 124 for some excellent books and Web sites.

BASIL: Basil does a whole lot more than just zest up a marinara! It can help with fatigue and depression, increase alertness, aid concentration, and relieve headaches, head congestion, migraines, and

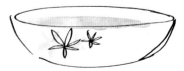

muscular aches. Try mixing this spicy, earthy smell with a citrus like tangerine or mandarin for a yummy scent.

BERGAMOT: This floral citrus scent is both uplifting and balancing and can fight stress-induced fatigue. While it can balance oily complexions, relieve skin irritations, and treat eczema, psoriasis, and acne, use it carefully in skin preparations.

CHAMOMILE: Chamomile is so relaxing that it's used in a lot of baby products. It can aid sleep, relaxation, and calmness. It can also be used as a mild astringent and it lightens and brightens blond hair.

CLARY SAGE: Relaxing when used in the bath, clary sage is also good when used in hair conditioner or as a mild astringent.

EUCALYPTUS: This distinctive, woodsy oil is exhilarating and works wonders on sore muscles.

Because of its cooling properties, it's a great addition to foot or leg products.

FRANKINCENSE: Wise men (and women) know this is a wonderful oil for meditation and spiritual practices. For your spa party, use it in treatments to calm the mind and soothe the spirit.

GINGER: Ginger can aid in relaxation and alleviate muscle soreness. Can irritate if not properly diluted.

GRAPEFRUIT: Mmm. This clean, uplifting scent can help treat mood swings, anger, depression, and stress. Grapefruit is a good astringent for balancing oily skin and hair, and it makes a good toner.

JASMINE: Use this rich, sweet, aromatic oil for your most sensual formulations. This pricey oil can be used to cleanse and soothe the skin.

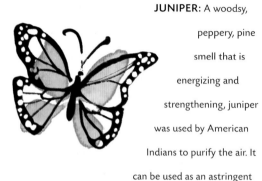

JUNIPER: A woodsy, peppery, pine smell that is energizing and strengthening, juniper was used by American Indians to purify the air. It can be used as an astringent for the skin and hair, and its cool, refreshing properties make it ideal for aching feet.

LAVENDER: My all-time favorite scent, lavender is calming and soothing and reminds me of a more genteel era. Lavender can be used as a hair conditioner and can heal burns and wounds. A multipurpose essential oil, lavender can be used before bed to promote sweet dreams and restful sleep.

LEMON: Lemon's clean, invigorating scent can purify the air and stimulate the mind. The strong oil can act as an astringent for oily skin and hair, but use with caution.

LEMONGRASS: A stimulating, inspiring oil that increases alertness and concentration, and relieves fatigue and aching muscles. It can work as a cleanser or astringent for oily skin. Use with caution and in a highly diluted form.

LIME: Has the same properties as lemon.

MANDARIN: Mandarin has both calming and rejuvenating effects. It's a good toner for oily skin.

NEROLI: This floral citrus scent can calm anxiety and lift the spirits. It's a great oil for the face when mixed with jojoba oil, and this combination makes a great balancing treatment for the skin and hair.

PATCHOULI: An effective antidepressant and stress reliever, patchouli helps tighten pores and combat wrinkles. It regulates oily skin and dandruff and is used to treat acne, eczema, and psoriasis. In my experience, its strong scent can often mask body odor.

PEPPERMINT: The most invigorating of the essential oils, peppermint reduces mental fatigue and increases alertness. Use in foot scrubs or lotions to cool and soothe, and to treat athlete's foot or fungal problems. It can relieve headaches and indigestion and can even be used in a mouthwash.

PINE: While there are different types of pine essential oils, all stimulate the senses and soothe the skin. I love putting them in bath oils and shower gels for a zesty morning pick-me-up. Take caution when using, as these oils are very strong.

ROSE: Rose calms the mind and relieves depression. When used as an astringent, it can aid dry, maturing skin and wrinkles.

ROSEMARY: Rosemary's another great-smelling, multipurpose oil to keep on hand. Its smell will perk you right up. A mild astringent, it can control dandruff, oily scalps and skin, and even acne. It's great for aching muscles when used in the bath.

SAGE: An antiseptic astringent, sage can be used on oily skin when diluted. It can also be used in mouthwashes for oral care and throat infections.

SANDALWOOD: This fragrant oil is excellent for dry skin and hair.

SPEARMINT: Kissing cousin of peppermint, spearmint is an invigorating, bracing essential oil. It increases alertness and opens up the respiratory system.

SWEET ORANGE: Can you tell I love the citrus smells? Brightening, refreshing, sweet orange oil can relieve stress

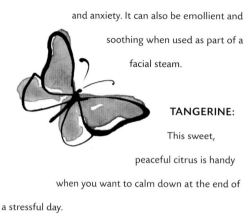

and anxiety. It can also be emollient and soothing when used as part of a facial steam.

TANGERINE: This sweet, peaceful citrus is handy when you want to calm down at the end of a stressful day.

TEA TREE: A top-notch antiseptic, tea tree oil works well when blended into foot scrubs or lotions. It's an extremely strong antifungal, antiviral, and antibacterial oil. Can be used in masks and toners to combat acne.

VANILLA: This familiar scent eases stress and invokes a feeling of comfort.

VERBENA: This oil has a lemony scent reminiscent of Pledge (and I mean that in a good way). Verbena can relieve depression, nausea, and sinus congestion. Do not use in skin care.

WINTERGREEN: Use this sweet, minty oil to revive and invigorate.

YLANG-YLANG: A sweet-smelling floral, ylang-ylang acts as an aphrodisiac, antidepressant, and spiritual balancer. While pricey, it can be used as a facial toner to balance oily skin.

TIP: Penny Ordway, founder of Philadelphia's Eviama Spa, recommends Dr. Haushka's Rose Body Oil. She calls the inexpensive but potent oil "pure love in a bottle."

TIPS FOR HANDLING AND USING ESSENTIAL OILS

✿ Always pay proper attention to the dosages of essential oils recommended on the bottle or in the spa recipe.

✿ Keep notes on blends or recipes you concoct so you can replicate your successes. Include ingredients and proportions, comments, and any ideas you may have on improving the product.

✿ Use only pure essential oils. You can generally find these at your local health food store.

✿ Handle with care and keep essential oils away from your eyes. And for goodness sake, do not ingest any oils. (Aromatherapists sometimes prescribe oral use, but unless you're one of these pros, do not swallow!) If you're a klutz, I'd recommend wearing gloves. If you get any oil on your skin or in your eyes, dilute it with vegetable oil immediately. If you get nauseous, feel dizzy, or have a headache from breathing in the oil, get some fresh air right away.

✿ Most essential oils should not be used undiluted on the skin. Try a patch test by diluting a few drops of an essential oil with a carrier oil and massaging it into the soles of your feet. Wash your hands immediately. If you don't have a reaction, the oil is most likely safe to use.

✿ Store bottles in a cool, dark place and keep bottles securely closed. It may seem obvious, but keep all essential oils away from children.

✿ Many essential oils lose their effectiveness as time passes or if they are not stored properly. Most have a shelf life of a year or more. Citrus oils have the shortest shelf life and should be used within a year; thick resins, woodsy scents, and "heavier" oils can improve with age.

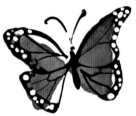

✿ If you are pregnant, stick to lavender and rose essential oils. Using other oils can be harmful. If you are

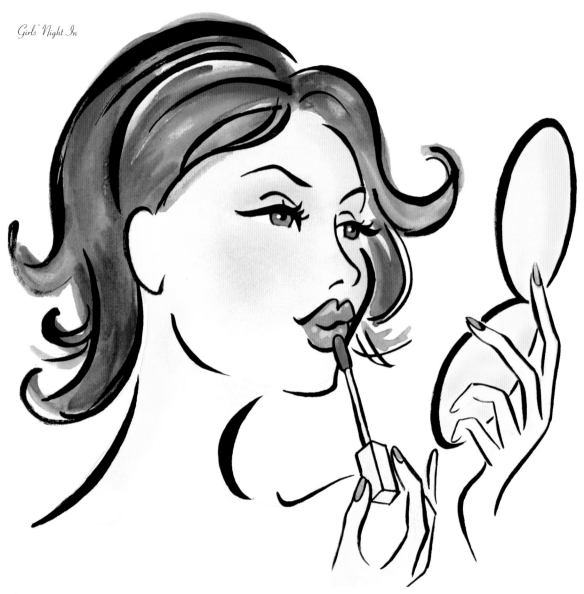

elderly or have a serious medical condition, do not use essential oils without thoroughly researching the individual oils first.

A FEW TIPS ON DILUTING

A good rule of thumb: the best dilution for most aromatherapy blends is 2 percent (that is, two drops of essential oil per one hundred drops of carrier oil). Going beyond a 3-percent dilution may actually cause adverse effects.

Here's a general guideline for use:

1-percent dilution: 5–6 drops essential oil per ounce of carrier oil

2-percent dilution: 7–14 drops essential oil per ounce of carrier oil

3-percent dilution: 15–18 drops essential oil per ounce of carrier oil

Packaging

Admit it. A new lip gloss, perfume, or moisturizer is always more appealing in creative or over-the-top packaging. But you probably have also learned the hard way that glass bottles in the shower are not a good idea. Or that you hate stuff in tubs—you'd rather have products come out nice and neat in a pump.

So first of all, when making products, make sure the packaging is functional and clean. Reuse old tubs and jars but sterilize them in a pot of boiling water before adding your treats. Look for fun plastic jars at art and craft stores. You can even use small paint jars for balms, lotions, and scrubs. There are many Web sites that offer packaging options (several are listed in the back of this book on page 124).

Label finished products with the date the product was made, ingredients, and instructions for use. Store any fruit or vegetable products in the refrigerator and use it within two weeks—or earlier if it looks suspect.

Setting the Spa Stage

While I give decorating tips for each spa, here are a few general suggestions.

MUSIC: Think soothing. You want tunes that can ease into the background and allow for maximum relaxation and distraction-free conversation. I like the following:

- Erakah Badu, *Baduizm*
- Kate Bush, *The Sensual World*
- Mary Chapin Carpenter, *Stones in the Road*
- Coldplay, *A Rush of Blood to the Head*
- Shawn Colvin, *Fat City*
- Alana Davis, *Blame It on Me*
  - Miles Davis, *Kind of Blue*
  - Stan Getz and Joao Gilberto, *Getz/Gilberto*
  - Sarah Harmer, *You Were Here*
  - Billie Holiday, *The Essential Billie Holiday: Songs of Lost Love*

- The Inkspots, *Java Jive*
- Norah Jones, *Come Away with Me*
- Lisa Loeb, *Firecracker*
- Lyle Lovett, *The Road to Ensenada*
- John Mayer, *Room for Squares*
- Sarah McLachlan, *Mirrorball*
- Natalie Merchant, *Tigerlily*
- *Midnight in the Garden of Good and Evil*, soundtrack
- Joni Mitchell, *Blue*
- Andrés Segovia, *The Art of Guitar*
- Van Morrison, *Moondance*
- Zero Seven, *Simple Things*

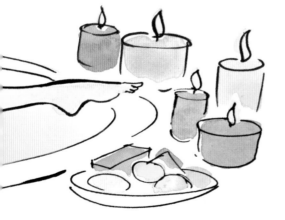

DECOR: Overhead lighting should be avoided. Instead, light candles and dim the lamps around the room. Keep lots of fluffy towels on hand. Throw cushy pillows on the floor for lounging. Clear clutter off tabletops and set supplies and snacks within easy reach of your guests.

CLOTHING: No matter what, guests should wear über-comfy clothing. Robes, pajamas, slippers, and sweats all get the spa stamp of approval. A simple rule of thumb: barefoot good, stiletto bad.

FOOD: Water, lots of it, should be on hand throughout the party. For some added zip, drop cucumber slices in one pitcher and slices of lemon, lime, or strawberries in another. Raw vegetables, herbal teas, fruit juices, and smoothies are also great spa staples. Your friends will feel healthy—inside and out.

PARTY FAVORS: Who doesn't like swag? While you may not be doling out expensive gift bags, it's always nice to treat your guests to a party favor or two. Something as simple as nail polish and an emery board can be an excellent take-home gift. A few other inexpensive favors are sure to please:

- Trial sizes of hand lotion, shampoo, and bath gel
- Shower caps
- Tweezers
- Lip balm
- Cuticle cream
- Headbands or hair elastics
- Copy of your favorite magazine
- Crystal or gemstone
- Travel containers
- A CD of soothing spa songs
- Comfy and colorful panties
- Dream pillow
- Essential oil blend
- Flowering plant
- Blank journal

GUEST LIST: You may just want to invite all of your favorite girlfriends over, but remember to take into account their compatibility. If you are tight with two women who don't get along with each other, it might be better to invite only one of them. Also, you only have so much space, time, and supplies, so make sure your home and planned treatments can accommodate your guest list.

The Ground Rules

Lay down the law when your guests arrive. Cell phones must be turned off. If you think a guest might sneak a call in the bathroom, confiscate all electronic equipment when they arrive.

❀ Trashy magazines can and should be read.

❀ Elastic waistbands are good; no waistbands are even better.

❀ Underwear is optional.

❀ Anything discussed or eaten during the course of the spa will go into the collective vault (i.e., what goes down at the spa stays at the spa).

- ✿ Guests are invited to bring their favorite body products, music, clothing, food, and booze.
- ✿ The day is about indulgence, fun, acceptance, and bonding. The day is not about guilt, competition, and self-restraint.
- ✿ Guests have to be willing to show themselves without a lick of makeup.

Every Day Is a Spa Party

Opportunities for spa treats are all around you. You can make any mundane event into a spa experience. To wit:

- ✿ If you're running errands, painting a wall, or helping a friend move, slather on a thick foot lotion (preferably with alpha hydroxy) and pull on some thick socks.
- ✿ If you've started a low-carb diet and you've got a half-used bag of granulated sugar lying around, put it to use on, not in, your body. While you're waiting for some water to boil, mix a little olive oil with a handful of sugar and exfoliate your hands and elbows.
- ✿ Stand on your toes or clench your buttocks while standing on the bus or train to work a few leg and butt muscles.
- ✿ Rub some cream (or even lip balm) into your cuticles while working at the keyboard.
- ✿ Put some oil, avocado, or deep conditioner into your hair and leave it in while you work out. Just pull your hair into a ponytail and add an old baseball cap.
- ✿ Light a candle at your desk (if it won't set off a smoke alarm).

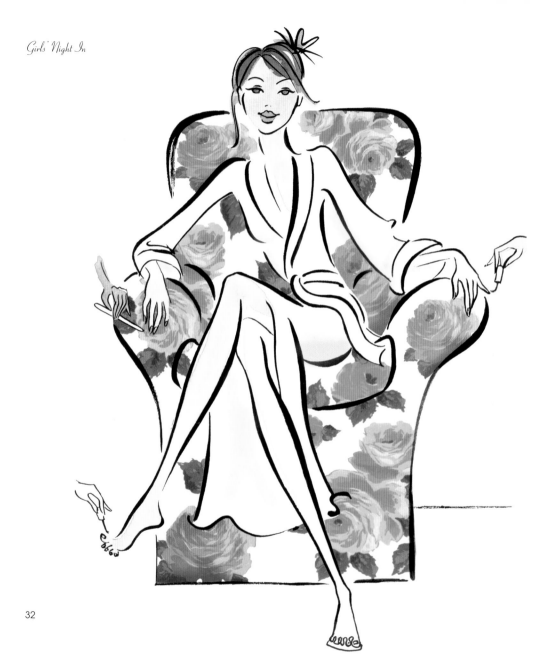

✿ Keep a rolling pin under your desk to massage your feet and arches.

✿ Pour your favorite essential oil into a dish or diffuser and let it scent your surroundings.

✿ Stretch whenever you're waiting in line. Stop short of the yoga position Downward-Facing Dog.

✿ If there's a break in a long meeting, close your eyes and focus on your breathing.

✿ Place an air-activated heat wrap on your shoulders to ease your muscles during your evening commute.

✿ Fill a clean sock with seeds or beans and a sprinkling of dried lavender. Knot the end and use it as a soothing eye or shoulder pillow during a flight.

✿ Add slices of lemon, lime, strawberries, or cucumber to your tap water.

✿ Washing dishes with hot water? Let the steam work its magic on your pores. Rub a bit of olive oil into your cuticles when done so your hands aren't dried out by the soapy water.

✿ If you're having a moment of writer's block, take your hands off the keyboard and give yourself a vigorous hand massage.

✿ Before bed, put an alpha-hydroxy lotion on your hands and cover them with old socks while you sleep.

Spring Spas

You know it's that time of year when:

- ❀ Flowers are blooming.

- ❀ Your allergies are flaring up.

- ❀ It won't stop raining.

- ❀ You want to wear strappy sandals but it's still too cold—and it won't stop raining.

- ❀ The air smells amazing—especially after a rainstorm.

- ❀ You swap your winter coat for a sassy slicker.

- ❀ You start exercising with renewed zeal, as swimsuit weather is just around the corner.

- ❀ You actually want to be outside.

- ❀ You paint your toes a cheerful shade of pink.

- ❀ You breathe. And you're dying to shed your winter skin.

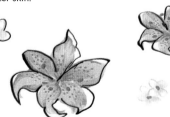

Spring is in the air, and boy, look what the air has done to your skin! After months of dry heat and frigid weather, your skin needs to be awakened, just like the crocuses and daffodils in your garden. If you're anything like me, you've probably hunkered down and treated yourself to warm baths and thick socks during the winter months. Even so, you probably blew your nose until it was red and raw and you looked like W. C. Fields (without the top hat, of course).

Spring offers a panoply of fresh ingredients to eat and incorporate into decadent body products. Papaya, pineapple, and other fruits are full of enzymes that can brighten and smooth the skin (fruit acid is a natural exfoliant). Milk, honey, avocado, and bananas moisturize the hair, face, and body. And oatmeal and sea salt can smooth rough skin. So feel free to try these ingredients on their own or in the recipes I've included here. Obviously, if you have an allergy, stay away from that

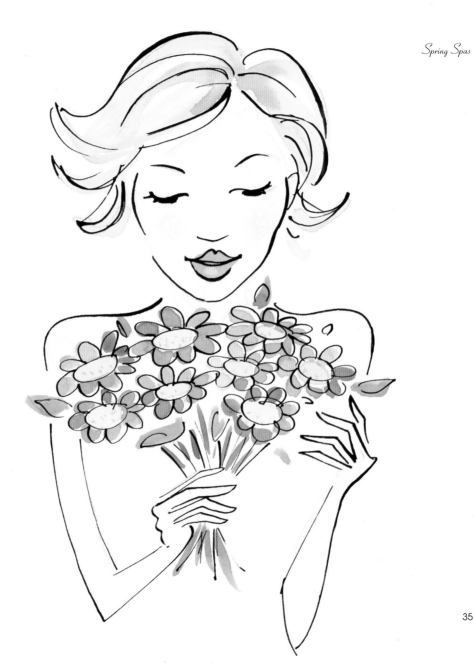

fruit or vegetable altogether. You don't want your fresh strawberry mask to induce an allergic reaction!

When you are decorating for your spa, incorporate items from the season. For spring, think fresh, bright flowers—potted plants make excellent party favors after they've brightened up your home spa—but also think outside of the box.

Buy rolls of floral wrapping paper and cover tabletops with it. Cut buds and float them in clear glasses of water. Give each guest a flower to tuck behind her ear as she walks in.

There are lots of reasons to celebrate spring. Here are a few ideas to kick-start your own creative juices:

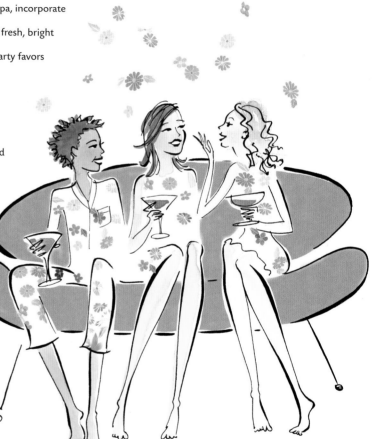

APRIL SHOWERS: Turn a rainy day into an excuse to stay in with your gal pals. Arm your guests with shower caps and send them one by one into your bathroom for the shower of a lifetime. Stock your bath with scrubs, shower gels, disposable razors, oils, lotions, and fluffy towels. While you wait for each guest to emerge from the steamy bathroom, play a classic board game like Clue or Scrabble.

TAX DAY: Get a great return on your investment . . . in your friends. Ask your pals over to collectively breathe a sigh of relief that the tax forms are in the mail. Trade shoulder massages or rub your guests' temples while they dream of financial success. Give them a few lottery tickets and a fun change purse to save their pennies in.

MAY DAY: You don't have to create a maypole to welcome the season with a joyful dance. Invite some friends over, put on some energizing music (I like Beyoncé's *Dangerously in Love* or the *Flashdance* soundtrack, but that's just me), and get down while lifting your spirits. Cool off with some refreshing cocktails, such as mai tais or frozen daiquiris.

EARTH DAY: Invite your friends over to plant your garden. After all the work is done, treat them to hand exfoliation, massages, and manicures, not to mention some lemonade and veggie treats. Send them home with a collection of seed packets.

MOTHER'S DAY: Invite all mothers over and hire a babysitter to watch the kids while you treat your friends to some pedicures and Bahama mamas. Have fun toys and snacks on hand for kids and adults alike. Feel free to play Mother May I?, as long as your guests only ask questions that revolve around spa pampering!

Energizer Spa

Rev up your engines in this reviving spa. Shake off the sleepy days of winter and get ready to bloom.

Don't worry about being a bit cheesy, this day is about getting down, getting jiggy, or getting just plain crazy. Energy is the word of the day, and guests should be ready to leave the lethargy of winter behind them in this invigorating spa.

First of all, set the stage for optimum oomph. Open all the curtains and crack the windows if it's warm enough. Fresh air is incredibly energizing. Put a reviving essential oil like peppermint or tangerine in a small dish and set it on the windowsill to infuse the room and give each guest an added boost with every breath.

Decorate the room in which you're hosting the spa with bright primary colors. Reds, oranges, and yellows are particularly stimulating. Fill bowls or vases with red apples, oranges, lemons, and even kumquats to serve as both eye candy and sweet snacks. A bouquet of gerbera daisies will add even more visual pop to the party.

Rather than soothing sounds of waves crashing against rocks, your songs should be selected for their ability to get your guests groovin', whether they want to or not. Disco tunes are guaranteed bootie shakers, as are guilty-pleasure songs from the eighties. Encourage your guests to show off their favorite dance moves. And as the hostess, you have to be willing to lead the way on this one, even if it means a conga line.

And when your guests are fully charged up, send them home with a bottle of multivitamins and a box of peppermint tea to keep them revved up all spring long.

Energizing Spinach Salad

My friend Laurel introduced this glorious salad during a girls' weekend getaway. All other salads are dead to me.

  1 bag baby spinach, rinsed and stems
      removed
  ¼ cup red onion, chopped
  1 Granny Smith apple, cut into thin slices
  1 tablespoon walnuts, chopped
  ¼ cup goat cheese, crumbled
  ¼ cup croutons
  dressing of your choice (I suggest a
      champagne vinaigrette)
  freshly ground black pepper

Mix everything but the goat cheese, croutons, and dressing and put it in the fridge. Add remaining ingredients and mix well when ready to serve. Add fresh pepper to taste.

YIELD: Serves 4 to 6

Peppermint Salt Bath

This bath is soothing to the muscles and uplifting to the spirit. Peppermint, in any form, will increase alertness and elevate your mood. What's not to like?

  ½ cup Epsom salt
  ½ cup sea salt
  10 drops peppermint essential oil (or
      substitute 1 peppermint tea bag)

Mix the salts together and add the peppermint oil. If you use a tea bag instead, mix the salts together and add a tea bag to the tub as you're drawing a bath. Store in a plastic or glass jar.

USAGE: Scoop a fourth of the mixture under running water and send your friends one at time into the bath for forced rejuvenation. You can also make up a jar of the salts for your friends as a party favor.

YIELD: 4 baths

TIP: Brush your body every day. Find a brush with natural bristles, and when your body is dry, brush your skin lightly, always up toward your heart. Try doing this before you shower or bathe. This dry, lymphatic brushing is a great energy booster and lightly exfoliates your skin.

Basil-Mandarin Massage & Manicure

Your guests will change their wills when you treat them to this three-in-one treat: the hand bath will perk them up, the massage will turn them to putty, and the manicure will make them look as good on the outside as they feel inside.

  5 drops basil essential oil

  5 drops mandarin
     essential oil

Emery board

Lotion

Cotton balls

Nail polish remover

Orange stick (a smooth stick with an
     angled edge used for manicures)

Clear nail polish

Nail polish (try a red-hot shade)

Lay a towel on a narrow table and sit across from your friend. Fill a small bowl with warm water and the basil and mandarin essential oils, and place her fingertips in it. After a few minutes, remove one hand and pat it dry. We'll skip the cuticle-removal stage, as that's best left to the professionals. Shape each nail with an emery board. The best shape to prevent breakage is generally straight across and slightly rounded at the edges. Once the nails are nicely shaped, put a dollop of lotion on her hand and begin your massage. You can add a drop of each essential oil to the lotion to further the aromatherapy benefits of the massage.

Here are a few basic reflexology hand-massage techniques from Michelle Ebbin, a Los Angeles-based massage therapist and the author of *Hands on Feet* and *Hands on Baby Massage*, and founder of Basic Knead (www.basicknead.com):

Hold her hand with both hands and simply apply precise pressure with your thumb all over her hand. Press firmly for about three seconds and then move to the next area. Press for a few seconds, and then make small, circular motions. If your friend flinches at any point, ask her to breathe deeply; spend a bit more time working that area. Pay special attention to the fleshy area between the thumb and index finger. Massage each finger, as well as between them. Press each fingertip for several seconds and release. End with an overall stroking of the hand and wrist.

Remove her other hand from the soapy water. Repeat the process.

When both hands are massaged, dip a cotton ball in nail polish remover and wipe each fingernail clean. Now you know the drill. Carefully apply a base coat, two coats of color, and then a clear top coat. Clean up any mistakes with the orange stick. Wrap a bit of cotton around the tip, dab it in nail polish remover, and run it over the cuticle until the polish disappears. Dunk her nails into a bowl of cold water for a few minutes to harden the polish.

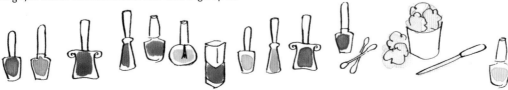

Urban Renewal Spa

This spa is for the professional or aspiring glamour puss. Shun the trendy and spendy spas of the big city and invite your downtown divas over for the glam slam of spas!

Let minimalism rule the roost in both clothing and decor. Pull your hair back, don sleek black tees and tights, and swipe on red lipstick. With your pale (that is, creamy) skin of winter, you'll be quite the drama mama. Ask all your guests to wear black to the party as well. Treat them to a makeover if you have a steady hand and a large beauty booty. Do your best to break them out of a style rut and introduce them to a new color or technique you've always thought would suit them.

Hide your clutter and place a few votive candles and clear glasses with rocks or lucky bamboo around the room. Lay out yoga mats for guests to stretch out on (very Gwyneth!). Soothe work-weary spirits with cool, dreamy music like *Simple Things* by Zero Seven. Send your friends home with a black cosmetic bag stuffed with a small mirror, black hair elastics, a red lipstick or nail polish, and the latest copy of *Vogue*. After a respite from the dog-eat-dog world out there, they'll be ready to strap on their stilettos and take the urban jungle by storm once again.

Cranberry Spritzer

While it may not be a cocktail, this zesty drink is great for hydration (and cranberry helps cleanse your urinary tract). I seek out 100-percent cranberry juice for maximum benefit.

½ cup seltzer water

2 tablespoons cranberry juice

3 frozen cranberries

Mix water and juice together. Serve in a

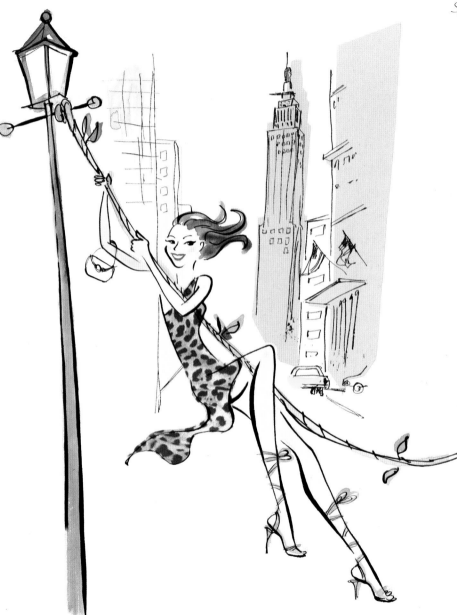

martini glass and drop frozen cranberries into the drink or skewer on a cocktail toothpick for that extra spa sophistication.

YIELD: 1 drink

Strawberry Face Mash

Strawberries are tasty in cocktails and fruit salads, but they can also be an effective skin treatment—they contain enzymes that are useful in getting rid of dead skin. Make sure you aren't allergic to this mask by doing a patch test on your wrist before applying the mash to your face. Great for oily skin.

1 large ripe strawberry

1 teaspoon honey

1 to 3 tablespoons powdered milk

Mash the strawberry in a small bowl or food processor until pureed. Add honey and enough milk powder to turn the mixture into a thick paste.

USAGE: Pull back hair and smooth a thin layer on your face. Leave on until it dries and you feel your pores tighten. Rinse with cool water and follow up with your favorite moisturizer.

YIELD: 4 treatments

Strumpet Lip Gloss

This lip gloss feels great, looks great, and smells great. You'll want to store one in every purse, pocket, or drawer.

- 8 teaspoons sweet almond oil
- 2 teaspoons beeswax
- 2 teaspoons cocoa butter
- 2 teaspoons honey
- 3 drops peppermint essential oil
- 3 drops lavender essential oil
- 3 drops rosemary essential oil
- Sliver of red lipstick or ⅛ teaspoon red mica powder
- 1 capsule vitamin E oil

PREP: Sterilize six empty lip balm tubes or containers by washing them with soap and water and then boiling them. Allow them to dry.

Put the sweet almond oil, beeswax, and cocoa butter in a double boiler (in a pinch, you can put the ingredients in a glass measuring cup and place it in a pot of water). When the water boils, turn down the heat to medium. Stir occasionally until everything is melted. Remove from heat and stir while the mixture thickens. Before the mixture completely hardens, stir in the honey, essential oils, and coloring. Puncture the vitamin E capsule and squeeze the oil into the mixture. Mix gently but thoroughly and pour carefully into containers. Allow to cool.

USAGE: Swipe on lips and kiss with abandon.

YIELD: Four ¼-ounce containers

NOTE: Experiment with other colors (dig out the remnants from your favorite tube of lipstick) or forgo the coloring if you just want an everyday, wear-anywhere gloss.

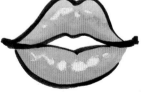

45

The Face Case

Looking for a new look? Think one of your friends is stuck in a rut with a serious mullet or thick glasses? Use your spa party as an opportunity to explore new looks. Pull out a pile of fashion and beauty magazines for inspiration. And don't just pick out hairdos or specs you like, pick out styles that look good on face shapes that match yours.

OVAL

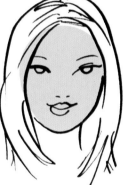

Hair: Those with an oval face can pretty much wear any hairstyle with élan. So rather than face shape, you can decide which feature (mouth or eyes, for example) that you want to highlight and you can take into account your hair texture (wavy, straight, etc.).

Glasses: Again, you can probably wear many styles, so try some wide Jackie O. frames.

SQUARE

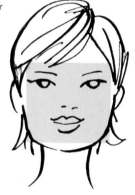

Hair: Soften the edges of a square-shaped face (i.e., a strong jaw) with soft bangs. Long hair should fall at least to the shoulders and short hair should be soft. In other words, embrace the round brush and beware the flat iron!

Glasses: Narrower frames with rounded edges will soften your face.

ROUND

Hair: To downplay your adorable chipmunk cheeks, go for sleekness on the sides and some lift in the crown. A shag or sleek bob (think Renée Zellweger) looks super and modern.

Glasses: To counteract your round face, opt for narrow frames with sharp, angular lines. Rectangular plastic frames would look great.

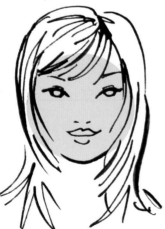

DIAMOND

Hair: To balance a narrow chin, which can look a bit severe, try a rounded shape with some fullness at the jawline, such as a bouncy, graduated, chin-length bob.

Glasses: If you've got high cheekbones, pick narrow frames that don't compete with them. Pick wide frames if the widest part of your face is lower and the area around your eyes is narrow.

PEAR

Hair: The opposite of diamond, you want to try to create fullness at the crown to offset a wider jaw. Layers are great for pear-shaped faces. Shags are super for short hair; if your hair is long, try a low ponytail or bun.

Glasses: Try on wider frames with sharp angles to even out your facial proportions.

HEART

Hair: Heart-shaped faces look great framed by a softer, curlier, chin-length style. Your objective is to create width around a narrow chin.

Glasses: Delicate, narrow frames look lovely on the heart-shaped face.

OBLONG

Hair: If you have a very long and square face, opt for width and volume. In other words, hair that's big—Farrah-big! Bangs can also help visually shorten the face if they hit at the brow.

Glasses: Add width with your glasses by picking frames that are thick plastic or even have varying colors at the temples.

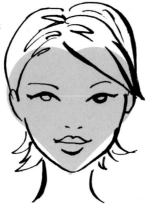

Coming-out Party

If you've got a hankering for the slow Southern life, this spa is right up your alley. Channel your inner debutante and instead of tiaras, give your friends sparkly headbands to keep their hair out of the way when they indulge themselves in this steamy spa.

For decorations, think pink and froufrou, like a fifties party bomb exploded. Fill the room with pink balloons, stick a few pink flamingos around, and crown the queen of the coming-out spa with a cheap tiara. Play music softly in the background (I love the soundtrack to *Midnight in the Garden of Good and Evil*, which features Johnny Mercer tunes), and set out card tables for bridge, pinochle, or gin rummy.

Serve guests mint juleps (or just spring water with a sprig of fresh mint) and shrimp cocktail. Place dishes of nuts, olives, and baby gherkins around the room for casual snacking. And don't forget to give these debutantes a special gift, be it a girly pair of underpants, a huge cubic zirconia cocktail ring, pink sparkly lipstick, or a book about those Southern women with wills of steel (*Gone with the Wind* or *The Divine Secrets of the Ya-Ya Sisterhood*, perhaps?).

Since the theme revolves around coming out, ask your guests a few questions about their own coming-outs:

✿ Did they ever pop out of their clothing?

✿ When did they feel most like a debutante?

✿ Share prom experiences and other firsts: first date, first kiss, first love, first day on the job, first facial/makeover/massage/manicure, etc.

Without further ado, let's shed your winter skin and get scrubbed and rubbed for the new party season.

Mint Iced Tea

What's better on a hot, lazy day than the cool taste of mint iced tea?

6 peppermint tea bags

Sugar to taste

Fresh mint leaves

Fill a large kettle with fresh, cold water and bring to a boil. To brew your tea, rinse out a teapot with hot water. Add tea bags. One bag yields two cups of tea. (When making iced tea, you should add one extra bag.) Pour in boiling water. Steep for 3 to 5 minutes and pour into a tall pitcher. Add sugar to taste. Serve over ice and garnish with fresh mint leaves.

YIELD: Serves 10

TIP: Make iced tea cubes. Just freeze some of the tea in an ice cube tray. Plop a couple into your guests' iced tea and really wow them with your hostessing skills.

Body Blaster Scrub

There's no better way to come out of your shell than to scrub that cold weather right out of your skin. This simple recipe will slough off dead skin while moisturizing at the same time.

¾ cup fine sea salt

1 tablespoon jojoba oil

2 tablespoons sweet almond oil

20 drops orange blossom oil

With a metal spoon, mix ingredients together in a small bowl. Scoop into a glass or plastic jar. Enjoy!

USAGE: Rub gently onto dry skin, paying particular attention to your elbows and feet. And OK, yes, rub it on your bottom while you're at it. Avoid contact with open wounds. Stand there and let the oils do their work for a couple of minutes. Turn on the shower and rinse, but do not soap up. Let the residual oil continue to moisturize your body all day long. Follow up with Butt Balm if you are feeling particularly indulgent.

NOTE: You can substitute peppermint, lavender, and rosemary essential oils, or any combination thereof. Do not add more than twenty drops of essential oil to the mixture.

YIELD: One 8-ounce tub of yumminess

TIP: Jacquelyn Overcash, founder of Get Fresh, is a firm believer in exfoliation. If you can't get your hands on her yummy Look Better Naked kit (which includes a scrub, body facial, and body butter), just brush your body with a soft, dry brush before you shower. My body tingles after I give it a good brushing. Always brush toward your heart.

Butt Balm

Your booty isn't the only body part that can enjoy this emollient treatment. Rub it in anywhere that feels dry, chapped, or just a bit rough. It's particularly effective on any recently waxed or shaved nether regions of your body.

2 teaspoons nonpetroleum jelly

2 teaspoons cocoa butter

2 tablespoons carrier oil, such as grapeseed
   or jojoba

2 drops orange blossom essential oil

Heat the nonpetroleum jelly, cocoa butter, and carrier oil in a double boiler over medium heat (if you don't have one of these, you can use a glass measuring cup in a pan of water). When the cocoa butter melts, remove from heat. Stir slowly until the mixture cools. When it thickens, add the essential oil and beat until

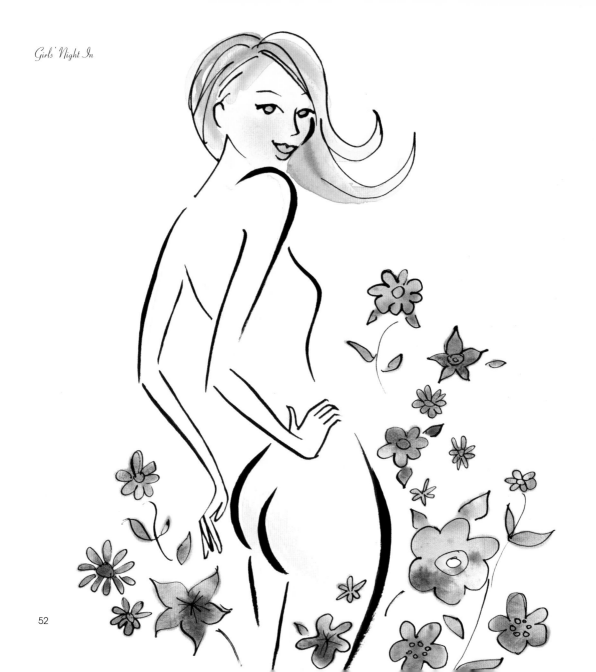

thick and creamy. Scoop into a clean jar and use as needed.

YIELD: Four ½-ounce jars or 8 applications

Cuticle Cream

This moisturizing cream can also double as a lip balm.

1 tablespoon beeswax

1 tablespoon shea butter

1 tablespoon jojoba oil or sweet almond oil

1 capsule vitamin E oil

8 drops lemon essential oil

Melt the beeswax and shea butter in a double boiler or in a glass measuring cup in a pan of boiling water. Add the jojoba or sweet almond oil. When all the ingredients are melted, remove from heat. Puncture the vitamin E capsule and stir it into the mixture. Add the lemon essential oil. Mix gently. Pour carefully into jars. Wait

for the cream to firm up before putting the lids on the jars or moving them.

USAGE: Rub a small amount into your cuticles whenever they are dry or ragged.

YIELD: Four ½-ounce jars

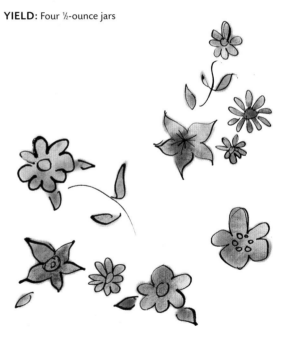

Summer Spas

You know you've hit June, July, and August when:

❀ You get a lot of sun, whether you want to or not.

❀ You sweat a lot, whether you want to or not.

❀ Hot dogs replace strawberries as your favorite food.

❀ You travel to destinations where conditions (i.e., plumbing) are often unknown.

❀ You take a road trip and enjoy the journey as much as the destination.

❀ You read a lot of trashy novels . . . for the third time.

❀ You suddenly develop an obsession with shimmery peach lip gloss.

❀ Inexplicably, your hair looks good when air-dried.

❀ SPF becomes a more important acronym than GC (gift card, silly!).

❀ You bare your skin—a lot of it.

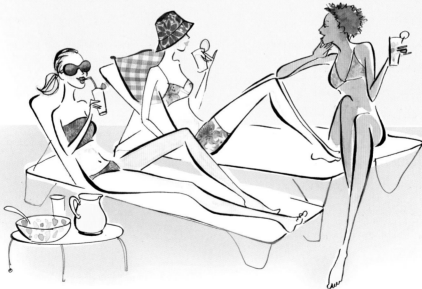

Summer means sunshine! And beaches, barbecues, beer, and bronzed babes, of course. All that time spent outside can be hard on your face, skin, and hair (and maybe your liver). You've been hearing about the importance of wearing sunscreen for years. But summer is also the time to eat lots of fresh produce and sweat through fun outdoor activities.

You might think that summer is a three-month-long spa in and of itself with all those weekend trips to the beach, but take time out to cleanse your skin and slow down your smokin' social schedule.

Host your spa parties outside if you can and soak up the sun-filled days of summer, since it's a proven fact that seasonal affective disorder goes into remission in the spring and summer months when the weather and our serotonin levels improve.

You can decorate with all the trappings of summer. Blow up a few beach balls and set them around the spa for a playful touch. Cover a table with blue sailcloth. Hand each guest a red or blue bandanna to tie her hair back for a patriotic touch. Set up a sandbox or wading pool in the backyard for guests to exfoliate or soak their feet, respectively. Flowers abound in summer, so make sure to place some fresh sunflowers or other cheery buds around the room.

Fruit and vegetables are also abundant during the summer months. While I highly recommend seeking out a fruit stand down a country road, you can also find fresh produce at your local supermarket. Discard your shopping list in favor of picking the vegetables and fruits that are most fresh when you cruise the produce aisle. What's better than fresh corn on the cob or Jersey tomatoes?

You could have an evening spa and grill vegetable and tofu kebabs and sip on blue Hawaiians or daiquiris. Oh, what am I saying? You can do this morning, noon, or night!

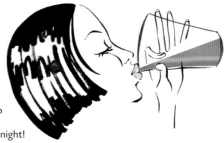

Don't be limited by the spas featured in this section. Here are just a few other ideas to jump-start your creative juices when cooking up a spa party.

SUMMER SOLSTICE: You don't have to be a pagan to celebrate the longest day of the year. Create wreaths out of flowers for each guest. Read horoscopes out loud. When the sun finally goes down, dance naked by the light of the moon and look for constellations in the night sky.

SCHOOL'S OUT FOR SUMMER: While you might not be subject to a teacher's dirty looks and piles of homework, summer is a time to celebrate throwing off the shackles of authority. Arm your friends with nonrequired reading (i.e., a juicy Judith Krantz or Patricia Cornwell paperback, or a stack of fashion mags) and spend the day doing absolutely nothing. Stretch like a cat, paint your nails, gossip, and watch classic teen comedies as you channel your inner teenager.

CELEBRATE YOUR INDEPENDENCE: Set the table with a patriotic tablecloth and serve up a picnic of lotions and potions. Put lotion infused with tangerine essential oil into a ketchup squeeze bottle. Fill empty pickle jars with a zesty salt scrub. Play horseshoes, croquet, or badminton while a cleansing clay mask goes to work on your face. Serve a mélange of fresh fruit on skewers.

LIFE'S A BEACH: If you can't go to the shore, bring the shore to you! Create a foot scrub with sand and a bit of oil to get your feet beach-beautiful. Comb a thick conditioner through your hair and let the sun's heat work the moisture into your hair. Load a cooler with a body spritzer, iced tea, snacks, and a cucumber you can slice and put on your eyes for a cooling treat. Fly kites, play volleyball, or just coat yourself with sunscreen and lounge around discussing hot men.

Camp Spa

No boys allowed! Revert to childhood, but instead of canoeing and telling ghost stories, pamper your guests and they'll be very happy campers. It has always been my dream to open a camp/spa for women. During their stay at this halcyon place, gals would learn new crafts such as knitting or jewelry-making in the morning (wearing their cowboy pajamas, of course), drink cocktails at lunch, take a class on kickboxing or sex toys (followed by a nap) in the afternoon, eat a big plate o' steak at dinner, and end the day by gossiping and eating s'mores around a campfire. Oh yeah, you'd also fit in some indulgent treatment like a hot stone massage into your day. Sounds downright dreamy, doesn't it?

Well, until I win the lottery, let's pretend that your apartment is really a log cabin and let's make camp!

Instead of childhood songs you used to sing on the bus, think about what you currently rock out to. Lead a rousing rendition of your favorite Madonna, Beyoncé, or Rolling Stones song to get your gals properly fired up. Of course, if you must sing something by Shaun Cassidy or the Bay City Rollers, I'm certainly not going to object!

Instruct the gals to wear their oldest, most comfortable T-shirts and shorts. Rips and paint splatters get extra points! In fact, give a prize to the guest with the rattiest clothing. May I suggest a box of Goo Goo Clusters or a copy of *Tiger Beat*?

And that brings us to the party favors. Try putting a care package together. Use a lunch box and fill it with nostalgic camp essentials: insect repellent, colorful bandages, blank postcards, bubble gum, a deck of cards, and a lanyard or leather keychain with their name on it. Throw in a few saucy contraband items, such as condoms, a bodice-ripper paperback, and fire-engine red nail polish, just to keep the little darlings on their toes.

And no self-respecting camp counselor would be caught without proper snacks. Fill a bowl with boxes of Cracker Jacks, packs of gum, and lollipops. Since this is a spa, temper the junk food with bowls of oranges, apples, and bananas. Cut up vegetables and serve with spinach dip. Throw a bag of ice in your sink and fill it with glass bottles of Grape Nehi and Orange Crush. Make Kool-Aid ice cubes and drop them into glasses of water for that extra zip.

For a more substantial dinner, wrap corn in tinfoil and cook it on the grill alongside some Polish sausages. As the coals are dying down, bust out the skewers and make s'mores. If you don't have a grill, you can toast some marshmallows carefully over a gas stovetop!

Spinach Dip

This is so addictive that whenever there's a party at my mom's house, I plant myself next to the dip so I can plow through it with whatever's handy. While it's delicious served in a bread bowl or with fresh bread, you can cut out the starches and replace the bread with vegetables.

1 package frozen chopped spinach, thawed
   and drained

1 package vegetable soup mix, dry

1 (16-ounce) container low-fat sour cream

1 cup low-fat mayonnaise

¼ cup chopped onion

¼ cup finely chopped carrots

¼ cup chopped hazelnuts

1 (8-ounce) can water chestnuts, drained
   and chopped

Mix all ingredients together and refrigerate for three

hours. Serve with slices of red, yellow, and green pepper,

baby carrots, celery stalks, or broccoli florets.

YIELD: Serves 8 to 10

Lemon Spritzer

This might sound like the newest cocktail at your local

nightclub, but although you can drink it, this body spray

is more refreshing on your skin. Think of it as a grown-

up, natural version of Jean Naté!

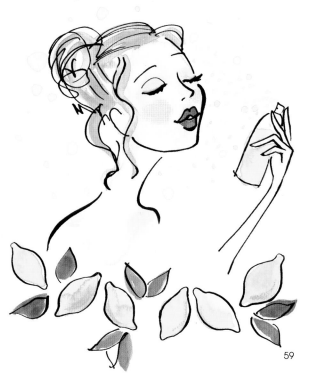

59

Juice of 1 lemon

1 cup distilled water

Sterilize a spray bottle (plastic hairspray pump bottles are perfect) in boiling water. When the bottle is dry, pour in the lemon juice and distilled water.

Shake well and spritz liberally all over your body. Pass it around the room so each guest can cool off with this pick-me-up, or have each guest make her own bottle to use and take home. Shake well before each use and keep refrigerated. Discard after two weeks.

YIELD: 1 cup

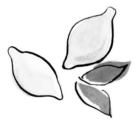

Face Painting Customized Masks

Here's a multitasking, grown-up version of face paint. There are masks to address every kind of skin type or problem. The most common kinds of skin are oily, dry, normal, and combination. Some women find that their T-zone is oily while the rest of their face is normal or dry. If that's the case, use the following colorful masks to treat specific areas of the face. Prep the skin by enjoying an aromatic facial steam before applying your mask.

GREEN WITH ENVY AVOCADO MASK

This is best for normal to dry skin.

1 ripe avocado

1 teaspoon to 1 tablespoon buttermilk

Peel and mash the avocado in a bowl. Add just enough buttermilk to form a paste.

USAGE: Apply to clean skin and leave on for 20 minutes. Rinse off and follow with a moisturizer.

YIELD: Good for 4 full-face applications

NOTE: This multipurpose mask can also be used as a deep-conditioning hair treatment.

PAPAYA DON'T PREACH MASK

This one is best for dull or oily skin.

   1 ripe papaya

Peel and remove the papaya seeds. Mash the fruit of the papaya in a bowl with a fork. Wrap a towel around your neck and pull your hair back.

USAGE: Apply a thin layer to clean skin. It will be runny, so be prepared. Kick back and gab while the papaya goes to work. Leave the mask on for 15 minutes

and rinse off with warm water. Finish up by applying a moisturizer.

YIELD: Good for 4 full-face applications

I CAN'T BELIEVE IT'S YOGURT . . . ON MY FACE

This simple white mask is great for blotchy skin, since it has mild bleaching properties.

   1 tablespoon plain yogurt

USAGE: Smooth the yogurt on a clean face and neck and allow to dry. Rinse and finish up by applying a moisturizer.

YIELD: 1 application

Granola Girl Spa

Turn even a high-maintenance mama into a nature girl in this earthy spa. Head for the great outdoors, whether it's deep in the woods or just a sunny spot in your favorite city park. Heck, host a spa in your backyard, if you've got the room. Just bring along sunscreen, blankets, and plenty of water.

Natural fibers are a must, so instruct your ladies to wear comfy linen or cotton clothing. As this is about getting in touch with nature, tell them to leave their unmentionables in the lingerie drawer! Nothing should bind or constrict today.

Rather than turning on a stereo, let the sounds of nature work their healing magic on you. Sing together if you're particularly inspired and sound your barbaric yawp through your neighborhood. Snack on yogurt parfaits, exotic fruits, fresh salad, and good old raisins and peanuts.

Give your gals a yoga mat bag and fill it with the best nature has to

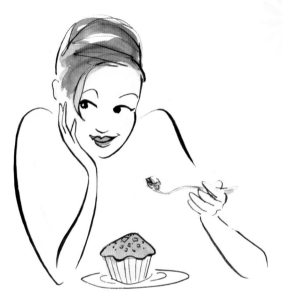

Perfect Yogurt Parfait

This is my favorite indulgent breakfast and it makes a great healthy spa snack.

    8-ounce container of nonfat vanilla yogurt

    2 tablespoons granola

    ¼ cup fresh berries

In a small, clear glass, layer half of your yogurt, granola, and berries. Repeat. Refrigerate until you are ready to serve. It's best to make this only a few hours before your party; otherwise, the granola can lose some of its crunch.

YIELD: 1 parfait

NOTE: You can add a sprinkling of wheat germ to the granola for added health benefits.

offer. Brad Pitt and Jude Law won't fit in the bag, so instead tuck fruits and veggies from the local farmers market in it, along with a plant or seed packets, organic honey, and even a jar of homemade jam you made ahead of time. They'll feel truly pampered and inspired.

The Classic Sun Salutation

This yoga sequence seems simple, but if you aren't careful you can get quite the head rush. So ease into the exercise and enjoy getting your body moving. Practice this prior to the party and stun your friends with your flexibility and peaceful demeanor as you lead them through this series of poses.

You can do this on any flat surface or, even better, on a yoga mat. Make sure your guests are spaced well apart so they don't bump each other during the exercise. While this should be done with fluidity of movement, be sure to breathe slowly and feel each stretch.

1.   Stand with both feet touching. Face in the direction of the sun. Bring your palms together at the heart.

2.   On your next inhale, raise your arms upward, keeping your palms together. Slowly bend backward, stretching your arms fully.

3.   Exhale slowly, bringing your hands out to your sides as you bend forward until your palms are on the ground.

Your hands should be alongside your feet, with your head touching your knees. If you can't do this, don't worry. Your guests probably can't either.

4.   Inhale. Take a large step backward with your right leg until you are in a deep lunge. Keep your hands and feet on the ground, with your left foot between your hands and your knee over your foot. Raise your head.

5.   While exhaling, move your left foot back so both feet are behind you, hip width apart. Keep your arms straight, raise your hips, and align your head with your arms, forming an upward arch. You are now in the Downward-Facing Dog pose.

6.   Inhale. Slowly lower your hips until they are slightly above the floor. Bend backward as much as possible.

7.   Exhale and lower your body to the ground until your feet, knees, hands, chest, and forehead are touching the ground.

8.   Inhale. Slowly raise your head and bend backward, arching your spine as much as possible. You should look like a cobra!

9. Exhale and raise your hips and align your head with your arms until you are once again in the Downward-Facing Dog pose.

10. Inhale, bend your left leg, and take a big step forward so that your left leg is between your hands. Lift your head up.

11. Exhale slowly and bend your right leg; bring it between your hands so that your hands and feet are aligned. Bring your head to your knees, if possible.

12. Inhale slowly and raise your arms out to your sides; sweep them slowly upward as you return to a standing position. Slowly bend backward, stretching your arms above your head. Return to position 1 and repeat the sequence once more—or several times, if you wish.

Almond Facial Milk

This gentle cleanser is ideal for dry, aging, and sensitive skin types, as it cleanses without stripping or drying the skin.

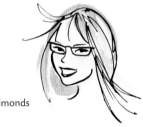

   ¼ cup whole milk

   3 tablespoons honey

   1 egg yolk

   1 tablespoon finely ground almonds

Put all the ingredients in a blender and mix for 1 minute at high speed.

USAGE: Spread cleanser onto your skin. Using a circular motion, massage it in with your fingertips. Wipe off with a tissue, or use a bit of water and a few cotton pads to rinse your face.

YIELD: 4 treatments

NOTE: Keeps for two to three days in the refrigerator.

Cleopatra's Milk and Honey Bath

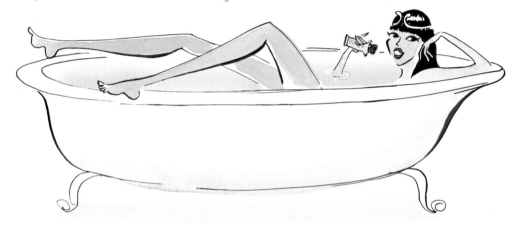

While you can't bathe outside, this is a lovely treat to give your friends to take home to continue the spa experience. This sensual treatment should encourage you to feel great about your naked body—every smooth inch of it!

- ¼ cup honey
- ¼ cup powdered milk
- 5 drops of your favorite essential oil (try rose, sandalwood, or ylang-ylang)

Mix all the ingredients together in a bowl and add to your bath.

USAGE: Dim the lights and slip into the royal waters. Unwind for at least 15 minutes. Gently blot your skin and take a couple of minutes to admire your naked form before rejoining the party.

YIELD: One to two baths

New Age, New You Spa

We are often scared of things that are unknown. Heck, a blind date can send you running for the hills. But relax—this day may involve palm reading, but no hand-holding! Today you are going to embrace all things "woo woo" in this mind-expanding spa. And if you like a regular dose of crystal therapy or Ayurvedic treatment, you'll even welcome the strange and unusual long after the spa is over. Opportunities are all around you to stretch your mind and body. Look into yoga classes at your gym, pick up a book on chakras or doshas, or buy a deck of tarot cards. Go ahead—it's fun to believe!

Ideally, you will host this spiritual spa in a backyard or secluded park. If you can manage an outdoor spa, make sure you have plenty of large blankets on hand (no one, no matter how earthy, likes grass stains on her knees!), sunscreen, bottles of water, lots of fruit and raw veggies, and even a few books on esoteric topics like palm reading, reiki, and crystal therapy.

If you're inside, clear out the room so you and your guests will have room for stretching, meditating, or lounging. Open the curtains and let the sun shine in. Light candles or incense and let the warmth of the sun and your friends work their magic on the spa. If you have a few extra minutes before the party begins, light a sage stick and wave it around the room. Focus your thoughts on what kind of good vibrations you want to generate at the party and your room will be prepared for a successful spa.

Send guests home with a crystal you've selected just for them. Place it in a small pouch. You could also give them a palm reading chart, a deck of tarot cards, a mendhi henna tattoo kit, or an essential oil blend customized to their Ayurvedic dosha. There are many excellent books on New Age topics; any one would be an enlightened choice for a party favor.

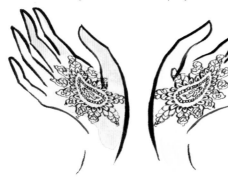

Caesar Salad with Lemon Dressing

This salad may sound boring, but the zesty low-cal, low-carb dressing transforms a classic into a spectacular spa dish.

1 head romaine lettuce, chopped

½ cup mushrooms, sliced

½ cup cherry tomatoes, halved

1 roasted chicken breast, diced

¼ cup Parmesan cheese, shredded

FOR DRESSING:

Juice of ½ lemon

2 anchovies (or 1 teaspoon anchovy paste)

2 cloves garlic, crushed

2 tablespoons olive oil

Fresh black pepper, to taste

Add all ingredients, except for the cheese, and toss. For the dressing, put all ingredients in a blender and mix until smooth and creamy. Pour over the salad, add the cheese, toss, and serve.

YIELD: Serves 4 to 6

Chakra the Monkey!

No, it's not a creature from *Land of the Lost!* "Chakra" is a Sanskrit term denoting one of seven major energy centers situated from the base of the spine to the crown of the head, plus scores of minor centers throughout the body. These correspond roughly to nerve clusters where nerves from every part of the body join the spinal cord. Many Indian and Chinese therapies, such as acupuncture, focus on reestablishing the free flow of energy throughout the chakras. When you weave the energies together, you achieve balance and wholeness.

The seven chakras are described on page 70. To activate each chakra, try placing the corresponding stone on the chakra, wearing or placing the corresponding color around your home, and scenting your body or room with the corresponding flower or fragrance.

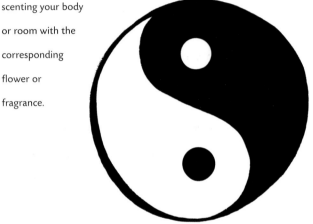

CHAKRA 1 (EARTH):
Located at the base of the spine, chakra 1, the root chakra, is associated with survival.

Color: red
Scent: cedar
Gemstones: lodestone, ruby, garnet, smoky quartz, obsidian, onyx, jet, hematite, bloodstone, red jasper

CHAKRA 2 (WATER):
Located in the lower abdomen, chakra 2, the sexual chakra, is connected to emotions and sexuality.

Color: orange
Scents: orris root, gardenia
Gemstones: carnelian, coral, agate

CHAKRA 3 (FIRE):
Located at the solar plexus, chakra 3, the personality chakra, is related to power and will.

Color: yellow
Scent: carnation
Gemstones: amber, topaz, citrine, tiger's eye

CHAKRA 4 (AIR):
Located just over the sternum, chakra 4, the heart chakra, is associated with love and balance.

Color: green
Scents: lavender, jasmine
Gemstones: emerald, peridot, tourmaline, rose quartz

CHAKRA 5 (SOUND):
Located at the throat, chakra 5, the expressive chakra, is connected to communication and creativity.

Color: blue
Scent: frankincense
Gemstones: turquoise, lapis lazuli, green aventurine

CHAKRA 6 (LIGHT):
Located at the center of the forehead, chakra 6, the knowledge or third-eye chakra, denotes intuition and imagination.

Color: indigo
Scents: mugwort, star anise
Gemstones: lapis, quartz, sodalite, blue sapphire

CHAKRA 7 (THOUGHT): Located at the top of head, chakra 7, the crown chakra, relates to knowledge and understanding.

Color: violet
Scent: lotus
Gemstones: amethyst, diamond, moss agate, white opal, moonstone

Pitta, Vata, and Kapha, Oh, My!

Ayurveda is a 5,000-year-old system of healing that originated in India. It translates as "the science of life" and incorporates cooking, nutrition, yoga, massage, meditation, and other body treatments. They all work to connect the body to the cosmos (as in the universe, not a boatload of pink cocktails).

There are three basic bioenergies—called "doshas"—in Ayurveda philosophy. Vata represents space and air and it regulates our energies and movements. Pitta represents fire and water and it offers warmth, perception, and the capacity to transform substances in our bodies. From water and earth come Kapha, which makes up our structure and flesh, and creates solidity and cohesiveness.

We all have differing amounts of each dosha in us. To determine your dosha combination, check out the quiz below. You can either photocopy quizzes for your guests or you can ask them the questions out loud. Once your guests identify which dosha sounds the most like them, ask each one to lie back; rub their temples or shoulders with an essential oil blend customized to their predominant dosha. Match the massage oil blends to each dosha. Use the Relaxing Blend for Vata, the Pick-Me-Up Blend for Kapha, and the Sensual Blend for Pitta.

I took this quiz while a guest at Mii Amo, a destination spa in Sedona, Arizona. It's a good way to get a basic understanding of your Ayurvedic constitution. For the record, I'm half Pitta, half Vata; I don't think there's a lick of Kapha in me.

Check off the most appropriate selection. For the more emotional and behavioral characteristics, answer according to how you've felt over the course of your lifetime, rather than over the past few months.

PHYSIQUE

- ☐ **A.** taller or shorter than average; light bone structure; protruding joints
- ☐ **B.** toned with an athletic body of medium height; medium bone structure
- ☐ **C.** stocky in build; tall and solid; heavy bone structure

WEIGHT

- ☐ **A.** thin and usually have been; thin as a child; difficult to gain weight
- ☐ **B.** well-proportioned frame; medium build as a child; gain or lose weight easily
- ☐ **C.** ample in build; was plump as a child; gain weight easily and have difficulty losing it

EYES

- ☐ **A.** small and/or narrow; active and dark
- ☐ **B.** a penetrating light green, gray, or blue; sensitive to light
- ☐ **C.** large and attractive, with thick eyelashes

HAIR

- ☐ **A.** dark; dry; wiry or kinky
- ☐ **B.** fine and light; blond, light brown, or red; may thin and gray early in life
- ☐ **C.** thick and wavy; a little oily; dark or light

COMPLEXION/TEMPERATURE

- ☐ **A.** a dark complexion and tan easily; dry skin that chaps easily; cold hands and feet; little perspiration
- ☐ **B.** fair and sunburn easily; can be oily; good circulation; generally warm; perspire easily
- ☐ **C.** thick, cool, and well lubricated; tan slowly and evenly; warm body; cold hands and feet; moderate perspiration

FACE
- [ ] **A.** long and thin; small features
- [ ] **B.** moderate size; angular features
- [ ] **C.** round and large; soft

PREFERRED CLIMATE
- [ ] **A.** a warm climate with sunshine and moisture; intolerant to cold, dry, and windy climates
- [ ] **B.** cool and well-ventilated places with fresh air; intolerant to hot and humid climates
- [ ] **C.** any climate, as long as it isn't too damp or humid; intolerant to cold, damp, and rainy climates

APPETITE
- [ ] **A.** variable; I can forget to eat; I like to snack or nibble; I like light foods
- [ ] **B.** very strong; I can become irritable if I miss a meal; I gravitate toward high-protein foods
- [ ] **C.** good; I'm okay if a meal is missed; I enjoy foods; I love fatty foods, breads, and starches

THIRST
- [ ] **A.** sometimes thirsty and sometimes not
- [ ] **B.** often thirsty
- [ ] **C.** rarely thirsty

DIGESTION

- ☐ **A.** okay; can become gaseous and constipated; stools can be hard and irregular
- ☐ **B.** excellent; tend toward heartburn and indigestion; stools are passed easily and regularly
- ☐ **C.** fine; may be a little slow; neither very regular nor irregular

SLEEP PATTERNS

- ☐ **A.** light or interrupted; 5–7 hours per night; lean toward insomnia
- ☐ **B.** very sound; 6–8 hours per night; fall asleep easily
- ☐ **C.** very deep; uninterrupted; have difficulty waking up

PULSE

- ☐ **A.** thin and rapid; light and variable; cold hands
- ☐ **B.** strong and full; bounding; warm hands
- ☐ **C.** steady and strong; slow and rhythmic; cool hands

ACTIVITY

- ☐ **A.** restless and fidgety; perform activities quickly; stay physically active
- ☐ **B.** competitive and perfectionistic; perform activities intensely and efficiently; enjoy activity
- ☐ **C.** leisurely in my activities; do things slowly, calmly, and deliberately

MENTAL ACTIVITY

- ☐ **A.** creative thinker with a quick mind; can change my mind easily
- ☐ **B.** precise, intelligent thinker with a discriminating mind; good initiator and leader; articulate
- ☐ **C.** detail-oriented thinker; good at keeping a project running smoothly; calm and patient

LEARNING PATTERN

- ☐ **A.** learn new things very quickly; I can forget easily if I don't write them down
- ☐ **B.** learn at a moderate pace after hearing new material two or three times
- ☐ **C.** learn things a bit slowly, but once learned, it is never forgotten

SOCIAL SITUATIONS

- ☐ **A.** lively and enthusiastic; can be nervous and insecure
- ☐ **B.** outgoing, assertive, and accessible around people; can be critical and impatient
- ☐ **C.** more of a listener than a talker

EMOTIONAL REACTION TO STRESS

- ☐ **A.** fearful, anxious, and worried
- ☐ **B.** angry, aggressive, irritable, demanding, and uncompromising
- ☐ **C.** complacent, steady, and calm; seek solutions; can become depressed

MENTAL TENDENCY

- [ ] **A.** questioning; theorize about the cause of events; creative; have changeable moods and ideas
- [ ] **B.** discriminating, suspicious, and judgmental; can be forceful about expressing ideas
- [ ] **C.** logical, stable, reasonable, and slow to judge or evaluate; steady, reliable, and calm moods

WORK HABITS

- [ ] **A.** selfless and often volunteer to help out
- [ ] **B.** work intensely, especially to achieve personal goals
- [ ] **C.** procrastinate; can take a long time to complete projects; very detail-oriented

ROUTINE

- [ ] **A.** enjoy spontaneity more than routine
- [ ] **B.** enjoy organizing and like routine, especially if I have created it
- [ ] **C.** enjoy working within routines and prefer it over spontaneity

FINANCIAL BEHAVIOR

- [ ] **A.** share money; spend it impulsively; can spend on trifles
- [ ] **B.** spend moderately and on special items to advance professionally; enjoy luxuries and gourmet meals
- [ ] **C.** save money; value quality purchases; spend freely on food and entertainment

DREAMS

- [ ] **A.** flying or running; searching; traveling; fear; I often do not remember my dreams
- [ ] **B.** passion; light; anger; jealousy; the sun; colors; I often remember my dreams
- [ ] **C.** romance; water or oceans; empathy or sadness; I remember dreams that seem significant to me

FORGIVENESS

- [ ] **A.** forgive and forget easily and often
- [ ] **B.** take a long time to forgive; can hold grudges
- [ ] **C.** understand that people make mistakes; rarely upset by others' mistakes

YOUR SCORE

- [ ] **A**s (Vata):

- [ ] **B**s (Pitta):

- [ ] **C**s (Kapha):

Vata

ELEMENTS: ETHER AND AIR

When in balance: active, alert, creative, slim, light and dry, excellent energy level, vital

When out of balance: fearful, nervous, anxious, insomniac, constipated

To balance Vata: Reduce cold and dry foods and excess protein. Eat whole grains, root vegetables, and soups. Stay warm and dry. Try to maintain a daily routine that includes regular meals and sleep patterns, and daily activities such as yoga, tai chi, nature walks, golfing, and occasional running.

Pitta

ELEMENT: FIRE

When in balance: intense, sharp, intelligent, confident, having a strong appetite and digestion, courageous

When out of balance: anger, jealousy, criticism, high blood pressure, heartburn, irregular body temperature, ulcers

To balance Pitta: Reduce hot and spicy foods, sour foods, and excessive alcohol. Eat salads, steamed vegetables, fruits, soybeans, tofu, and light beans. Remain calm and cool. Engage in physical activity during the cool or evening hours. Cool, quiet, contemplative activities, such as evening meditation, are excellent practices.

Kapha

ELEMENTS: WATER AND EARTH

When in balance: relaxed, calm, stable, affectionate, dependable, strong, understanding, patient

When out of balance: dull, lethargic, possessive, overweight, depressed, having sinus problems and slow digestion

To balance Kapha: Reduce dairy, ice cream, and fried foods. Eat light foods like salad, light beans, and seafood. Stay warm and dry and remain active. Try to avoid eating late and oversleeping. Engage in physical activities that stimulate: gardening, sports, spring and fall cleaning, vigorous massage.

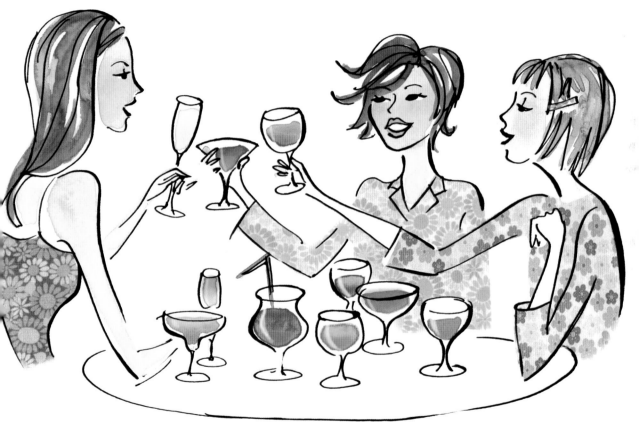

Autumn Spas

You know you've hit the fall season when:

✿ Leaves start changing color and falling to the ground.

✿ You go back to school.

✿ You give up open-toed shoes reluctantly.

✿ You suddenly have the urge to color your hair auburn.

✿ You hunker down and welcome the cold weather.

✿ Football games equal cute boys in tight pants.

✿ Halloween, Election Day, and Thanksgiving, oh my!

✿ You eat more—pies, for example.

✿ You start to close windows and doors to trap dry heat in the house.

There are few pleasures better than rolling around in a pile of leaves. Or drinking hot cocoa on a cool night. Or picking apples. Or better yet, bobbing for apples. Or even better, eating apple crisp. Mmm, apple crisp.

Autumn is a glorious season of color and comfort. It's my favorite because summer usually tuckers me out and I'm looking for any excuse to hunker down and wrap myself in a shawl (and to be honest, eat pie). And as the weather starts to get a bit, well, nippy, it's the perfect time to don your ex-boyfriend's sweater and your favorite jeans and kick back with your girlfriends.

Why not make it an autumnal spa party? It's harvest time and pumpkins and apples, not to mention wine, are in abundance. Serve up your favorite casserole, lasagna, or baked goods. Lighting is the key to setting a cozy mood, so dim the lights and lay a fire instead (throwing a few pinecones on the fire will infuse the room with a nice, woodsy smell). Sprinkle a few scented candles and large, fluffy pillows around the room. To really get into the spirit of the season, bowls of acorns, pinecones, and even leaves can create a feeling of warmth. A simmering pot of cinnamon-spiked cider will make your guests feel like they died and went to a wooded heaven.

As far as music, go classical. A bit of Brahms will go nicely with your Beaujolais. Ask your guests to wear shades of forest green, teal, burnt orange, and warm brown. Everything should be soothing to the eye and the spirit. And while fall is a great time for a girl gathering, there are a few specific events to which you might want to pay homage with a bit of spa pampering:

BACK TO SCHOOL: You may have graduated, but the scent of freshly sharpened pencils wafts through the air

every autumn. Ask a few friends over to follow along to a belly dancing, tai chi, or salsa dancing video. You're never too old to pick up a few new moves. Pull out your stash of makeup and perform glamorous makeovers on your girlfriends. As evening approaches, move the party to a dance club.

BREAST CANCER MONTH: October is National Breast Cancer Awareness Month in the United States, so take time to honor your boobs. Ask guests to come sans brassiere and indulge the décolletage: exfoliate with a body scrub and massage in an emollient lotion. Each guest will most likely want to do this to herself! Hand out pink ribbon pins and breast self-exam instructions as they leave.

ELECTION DAY: Gather your civic-minded friends for a trip to the polls, followed by a spa. Celebrate our democracy by voting on what movie, music, or cocktail to enjoy. In honor of our two-party system, give guests a choice between two face or body treatments. Toast to life, liberty, and the pursuit of happiness!

WINE: The Beaujolais is flowing, so gather your gals together to stain your teeth red while chilling with face masks and some Italian tunes. Whether it's Louis Prima or accordion music, toast to wine, women, and the pursuit of la dolce vita.

HALLOWEEN: Use the face masks in the Camp Spa party (see page 61) to create fun designs on this impish holiday. After doling out sweets to the neighborhood children, turn off your front-door light and hunker down behind closed curtains with bowls of your favorite chocolates, caramel apples, and spiked cider. Carve pumpkins (puree the pulp for a fresh enzyme mask) and reward the best design with a scented pillar candle.

THANKSGIVING: Sometimes single gals live just too far away to visit their families during the holidays, so invite your urban tribe over for an untraditional Thanksgiving. Cook a turkey and delegate appetizers, drinks, side dishes, and dessert to the guests. Definitely wear roomy pants, and when you're lolling about in a food coma after dinner, relax with foot massages, back rubs, or facials. Just stay away from the belly! Forgo party favors and just send each guest home with leftovers.

HAYRIDES: Take your girls for a drive or walk in the country. Stop to pick apples or check out the fresh produce and strapping farmhands at a farm stand. Be sure to breathe in as much country air as possible. When you return, bake an apple crisp, light a fire, tie a bandanna around your head, and slather on some Honey-Oatmeal Facial Scrub (see page 85).

Grandma's Kitchen

Autumn reminds us of bonfires, hot apple cider, and comforting smells wafting from the kitchen. Specifically, Grandma's kitchen. When the weather gets blustery and downright mean at times, Grandma's kitchen is always a source of joy and warmth. And yes, pie.

With very little effort, you can re-create that feeling of security and comfort in your own home spa. Dim the lights, light a fire or candles, and gather your friends around a big kitchen table. Lay out a tablecloth and put the ingredients for your spa recipes in colorful bowls.

Serve your guests warm apple crisp (the smell of the cinnamon will drive them crazy during the spa) with milk or coffee. Keep them hydrated with plenty of water, tea, or cider. They'll never want to leave.

In fact, don't be surprised if they call their parents for permission to stay over!

For a homespun party favor, give each gal a recipe box and fill it with a few of your favorite recipes, a book of crossword puzzles, a box of dominoes, and a farmer's almanac.

Your guests are in heaven and we haven't even mentioned the spa treatments, which might smell good enough to eat—but they do more good *on* your body than *in* your body.

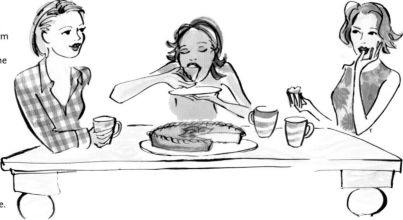

Cowboy Cookies

Forget about that Neiman Marcus urban legend cookie recipe. This recipe was handed down to me from my grandmother. After many years of happy experimentation, I think I've perfected the recipe and have never made another kind of cookie since.

2 sticks margarine, softened

1 cup white sugar

1 cup brown sugar

2 eggs

1 teaspoon vanilla

2 cups flour

1 teaspoon baking soda

½ teaspoon baking powder

2 cups oatmeal

1 package semisweet chocolate chips

½ cup nuts, optional

Preheat oven to 350°F. Beat together margarine, white sugar, brown sugar, eggs, and vanilla. Sift together flour, baking soda, and baking powder and add to the mixture. Fold in oatmeal, chocolate chips, and nuts if desired. Grease and sprinkle flour over a cookie sheet. Place balls of dough (about the size of table-tennis balls) two inches apart on the cookie sheet and bake for 8 minutes. Since many oven temperatures vary, keep an eye on your first batch. At the first hint of browning, take them out. They should be very soft and doughy. Carefully remove cookies with a spatula and allow to cool. Store in an airtight container to keep them soft. Serve with an ice-cold glass of milk. Dunking is encouraged!

YIELD: About 50 to 60 cookies

Honey-Oatmeal Facial Scrub

This exfoliating mask feels great, smells great, and is great for the skin. While the scrub is going to work on your face, relax and enjoy a nice cup of tea . . . with honey, of course.

  2 teaspoons pure honey

  1 teaspoon oatmeal

Mix the honey (don't eat it!) and oatmeal in a small bowl.

USAGE: Rub the goop onto your face in gentle, circular motions. Relax and let this decadent snack for the face go to work. Leave on for 10 minutes and rinse off with warm water. Follow up with your favorite moisturizer.

YIELD: 1 treatment

NOTE: Prep the skin by enjoying an aromatic facial steam before this treatment.

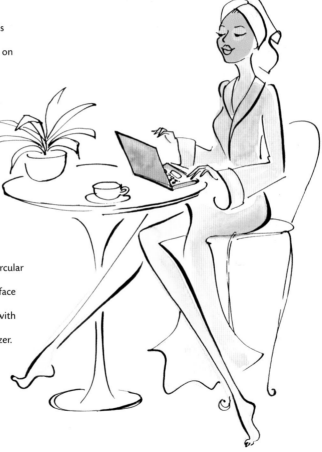

Tea-Bag Eye Soother

You can't really call this a "recipe," since it only involves some hot water and a couple of tea bags, but that's the beauty of this treatment. Multitask those tea bags—chamomile is a super soother, both inside and out.

    2 chamomile tea bags

Steep two bags in a cup of boiling water for several minutes. Put the cup of tea, along with the tea bags, in the refrigerator until cool.

USAGE: Use the chilled tea as a refreshing toner for the face. Just swipe on with a cotton ball. Close your eyes, lie back, and place the tea bags on your eyelids to calm the skin and the spirit. Tea keeps for a week if refrigerated.

YIELD: 1 cup of tea

Crème Brûlée Body Soufflé

After experimenting at length in my kitchen, I hit upon the creamiest, most luxurious cream known to woman. My friends went weak in the knees when I presented them with a pot of this dessert for the skin. And the best thing is that you'll become a delicacy for any man you like. If you thought vanilla reeled the boys in, try this!

    2 tablespoons cocoa butter

    ½ cup unscented body lotion or cream

    1 vitamin E capsule

    15 drops caramel fragrance oil

    15 drops milk chocolate fragrance oil

    1 teaspoon shimmer powder (or lipstick sliver,
        preferably in light gold or silver shade)

Melt cocoa butter over low heat in a double boiler or in a glass measuring cup in a pan of boiling water. In a small bowl, mix body lotion and vitamin E capsule. Quickly mix in the melted cocoa butter. Add fragrance oils and coloring (if you choose to tint your cream with a lipstick sliver, melt it with the cocoa butter in the double boiler). Once you've thoroughly mixed your ingredients, spoon the lotion into a plastic or glass jar.

USAGE: Slather all over your body and rub up against someone you like a lot. They will like you too!

YIELD: One 8-ounce jar

NOTE: You can substitute your favorite essential oil for the fragrance oils. You will just smell like an herb garden instead of a bakery.

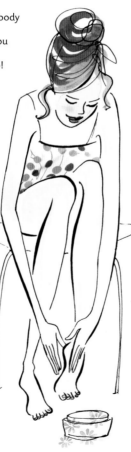

Lavender Linen Water

All the rage, traditional French linen waters can be used to mist clothes while ironing. During your spa, mist towels and curtains for a subtle, soothing scent.

> 1 teaspoon essential oil (lavender is customary, but you can also substitute your favorite)
>
> 2½ tablespoons vodka (100 proof)
>
> ½ cup distilled water

Combine the essential oil and vodka. Shake to blend. Add water. Store in a glass spray bottle and shake gently before using.

USAGE: Spritz on clothing before ironing.

YIELD: About ¾ cup

It's a Mood Point Spa

As the days get shorter, your mood can turn darker. Banish the blues in this uplifting aromatherapy and color-therapy spa. Make sure to have colorful drinks like cranberry juice or apple martinis on hand—that'll improve any toxic babe's temperament!

When decorating for your day spa, the important thing is to have color—joyous, riotous, ridiculous color—everywhere. Fill clear vases with bright flowers or oranges and apples, or even colored balls. Pick up a few yards of different colored fabrics and drape them over windows, tables, and even chair backs to perk up or calm down your guests. If you have enough space, set up one room as a restful oasis in greens and blues and set up another as a revitalizing room with hot colors like red, orange, and yellow dominating the color scheme. Ask guests to wear something in their favorite color or in which they just feel radiant.

After the spa, send your guests home with a package of food coloring and a box of crayons or paints so that they can color their world on a daily basis.

The Classic Cosmopolitan

I can't think of many things that elevate a mood quite like the rosy cheer of a cosmopolitan. Here's my favorite, compliments of my pal Brian (who shared the secret with me one night as we downed several drinks and gave each other facials).

2 ounces Absolut Mandarin vodka

½ ounce Cointreau

½ ounce lime juice (freshly squeezed, if possible)

½ ounce cranberry juice

Fresh lime to garnish

Mix ingredients in a shaker with ice. Pour into a martini glass and garnish with a twist of lime. For a yummy frozen version, mix ingredients with crushed ice in a blender. For a colorful twist, throw a few gummy bears into your drink.

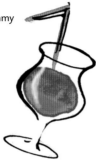

YIELD: 1 drink

COLOR THERAPY: A PRIMER

I once heard that warm colors like red and yellow stimulated the appetite. Hence, McDonald's and Burger King adopted these shades in their restaurant decor. If you want to relax (or maybe diet!), cooler hues of blue and green might do the trick. Color therapy is becoming more and more accepted in fields as diverse as alternative medicine and interior design. Spas use the basic principles of color therapy when designing their facilities, particularly their treatment rooms, and during select treatments. Check out page 90 for a basic primer on colors and their mood responses.

✿ *White:* Basis for all colors; strengthening, cleansing, nurturing, calming, purifying; promotes spirituality, vitality, and creativity

✿ *Red:* Stimulating, strengthening

✿ *Orange:* Revitalizing

✿ *Yellow:* Stimulating, awakening

✿ *Green:* Restful, revitalizing, balancing

✿ *Turquoise:* Restful, purifying

✿ *Blue:* Restful; promotes creativity

✿ *Indigo:* Restful, purifying

✿ *Violet:* Stimulating, purifying, transforming

✿ *Magenta:* Clearing; promotes spirituality

✿ *Pink:* Soothing; awakens compassion, love, and purity

✿ *Black:* Protective, grounding, calming; best when used with white or other colors

✿ *Gold:* Revitalizing, strengthening, amplifying

Many spa professionals believe in the power of color therapy to treat and ward off diseases. For example, use orange to stimulate lymphatic flow or imagine a yellow roof over your head to avoid sunburn and stave off ultraviolet rays.

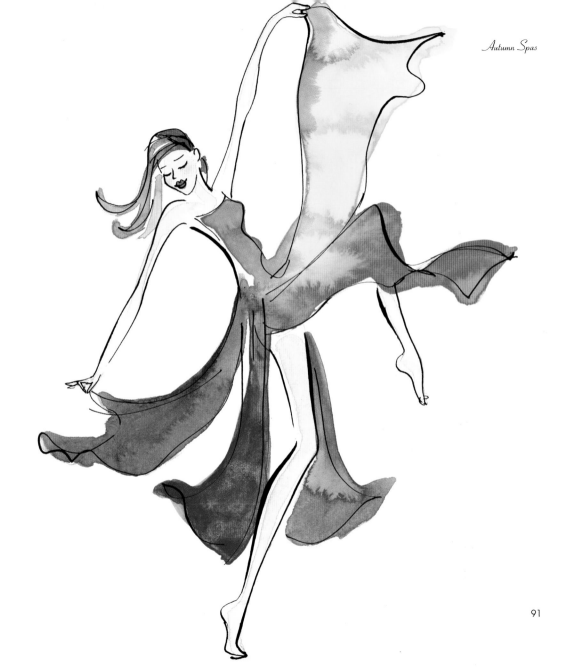

Herbal Pine Footbath

Stimulate your feet and your senses with this vibrant and moisturizing footbath.

1 basin filled with hot water

¼ teaspoon pine essential oil

10 drops green food coloring

1 tablespoon carrier oil

Mix all ingredients in a basin, bucket, or bathtub (you can fill a bathtub with hot water so that it covers your feet and ankles and sit on the tub's edge while you soak your feet).

USAGE: Dip your feet in and soak until your feet get pruney. Pat feet dry with a fluffy towel, slather with lotion (may I suggest another pine-scented product?), and put on some thick socks or paint your toes (refer to the color chart on page 90 to select a nail polish that matches your guest's intended mood).

YIELD: 1 footbath

NOTE: You can also add 10 to 15 drops of tea tree oil to increase the footbath's antiseptic properties.

The Zen Den

Things get serious and hectic in the fall as kids go back to school and workplaces get busy after the lazy days of summer. To counter the craziness, create a peaceful oasis in your home for yourself and your friends. You may not know quite how to meditate, but even the busiest career woman knows the benefits of taking a few minutes out to breathe in the company of her friends.

I look to the Far East for ideas on creating a calming, soothing environment. A friend of mine once told me that the four basic tenets of feng shui involve clearing half of your walls and surfaces; chucking anything cracked, chipped, or broken; making sure your doors—particularly your front door—are clean, painted, and in good working order (no squeaky hinges or faulty locks, please!); and, most importantly, loving everything you own. To that end, clear out a room. (It's unrealistic to expect you to clean out your spare closet or junk drawer, so just do the best you can in the room where you're hosting the party.) Oil the hinges on the front door and wash it down with some soap and water.

Using sand, a few rocks, and a small box, make a Zen garden on a tabletop and have your guests take turns creating shapes in the sand with a toothpick or fork. Set a few clear vases around the room with stalks of lucky bamboo. Fill pottery bowls with river rocks. Light tealights and place them around the room. Ask your guests to

93

wear clothing in neutral shades so that nothing distracts your eyes during the party.

Ply your guests with California rolls, edamame (soybeans), and green tea. When they reluctantly leave your Zen den, give them a small book on feng shui, a mini Zen garden or sushi kit, a lucky bamboo plant, or some incense.

California Rolls

This basic sushi recipe comes from my pal Alison Rooney, who brought a platter of California and avocado rolls to a spa party I threw last year.

6 tablespoons rice vinegar

2 tablespoons sugar

2 teaspoons salt

3 cups uncooked Japanese short- or medium-
    grain rice

3¼ cups water

5 sheets nori (dried seaweed)

1 large cucumber

2 to 3 avocados

½ pound imitation crabmeat

Wasabi (Japanese horseradish)

Soy sauce

Pickled ginger

In addition, you'll need:

Clean cutting board

Bamboo rolling mat

Plastic wrap

Sushi knife or very sharp knife

Soak rice in a bowl of cold water until it becomes cloudy. Rinse and repeat until the water is clear. Soak for an additional 30 minutes in water. Drain water and put rice in a pan with 3¼ cups cold water. Cover with a tight lid and cook on medium-high until water boils. You will see white foam oozing out from under the lid. Turn down the heat and simmer for 15 minutes. Turn off the heat and let the rice steam with lid on for 15 minutes.

Wash, peel, and remove seeds from the cucumber, and then cut into strips. Peel and quarter the avocados and cut into strips. Cut imitation crabmeat into—you guessed it—strips.

Combine the rice vinegar, sugar, and salt in a saucepan on low heat until the sugar dissolves. Drizzle over cooked rice and mix in thoroughly so that the rice becomes a bit sticky.

Lay out the bamboo rolling mat on a clean cutting board, cover the mat with plastic wrap, and place a sheet of nori, lengthwise and shiny side down, on top of it. Cover nori with a thin layer of rice, leaving ½ inch of space at the top. Add a strip of cucumber, crab, and avocado. Hold the filling in place with your fingers and roll up and away with your thumbs. Wet the

½-inch edge of nori with warm water and seal the roll. Wrap in plastic wrap and refrigerate until you are ready to eat. When you are ready to serve, remove wrap, wet a sharp knife, and cut the roll into pieces. Each roll produces six to eight pieces, depending on the thickness. Repeat the rolling process until you have enough pieces for your party. I suggest about six to ten pieces per guest, unless you have lots of other snacks on hand.

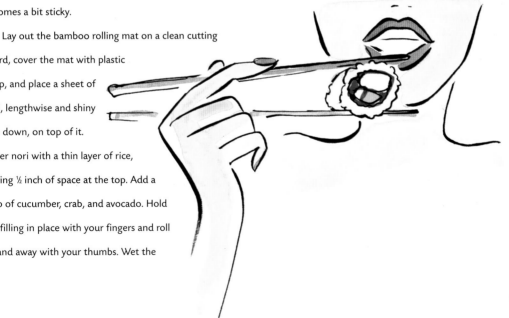

Serve with wasabi, soy sauce, and pickled ginger. Green tea and steamed edamame make a perfect accompaniment. Pass out chopsticks to each guest; they can wash them and reuse them as colorful hair accessories.

NOTE: A variety of other tasty ingredients can be used: mushrooms, asparagus, green beans, bell peppers, cooked shrimp, or sushi-grade tuna or salmon (just be careful about proper refrigeration and handling).

Hot Stone Massage

The most enjoyable and relaxing massage I've ever had involved hot stones and a hot masseuse named Vladmir. I can't help you with the guy, but I can help you with the stone massage.

4 large river rocks

1 ounce massage oil

8 small, flat pebbles (optional)

PREP: Prior to your party, collect the river rocks. This is a great excuse for an early morning trip to the beach (or the craft store). Rocks should be flat and about the size of your palm. Wash them thoroughly with soap and hot water.

Boil the rocks in a large pot of water. Let the water cool a bit. Make sure they aren't too hot or they'll burn the skin.

Instruct your friend to lie on her stomach on a bed, couch, or even the floor. Spread a sheet over her, and place a rock at the base of her spine, one at the middle of her back, and one on the sole of each foot. When the rocks cool, remove the sheet. Put a little bit of massage oil on the person's back and then use each rock as a tool, pressing the rock into the muscles. Use your hand to glide the stone up and around each muscle, avoiding the spine and any bony areas.

For a great treat for your guests (and yourself!), give them a hot stone foot massage. Using small pebbles heated in same way as the large stones, just focus on the feet. Place a stone between each toe and use one larger stone to press into the sole of the foot. You affect the whole body when you work on the feet. Just placing a stone between the big toe and second toe affects the brain.

TIP: Drink lots of water after a massage. If you want to detoxify, down some wheatgrass juice before and after your treatment.

TIP: Take advantage of the extra hands at the party and enlist a friend's help in applying a back facial or body wrap.

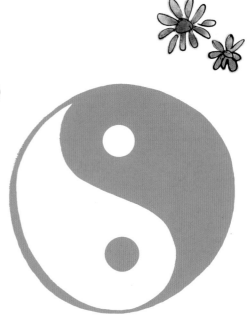

Massage Oils for Every Mood

These easy and effective massage oils come from massage therapist and author Michelle Ebbin. Pour all ingredients in a dark bottle and store in a cool, dark place. Shake well before each use.

RELAXING BLEND

⅔ cup grapeseed oil

⅓ cup wheat germ oil

10 drops vitamin E oil

8 drops lavender essential oil

8 drops chamomile essential oil

PICK-ME-UP BLEND

⅔ cup grapeseed oil

⅓ cup wheat germ oil

10 drops vitamin E oil

6 drops eucalyptus essential oil

4 drops rosemary essential oil

SENSUAL BLEND

⅔ cup grapeseed oil

⅓ cup wheat germ oil

10 drops vitamin E oil

6 drops sandalwood essential oil

4 drops bergamot essential oil

USAGE: Pour some oil in the palm of your hand and rub it between your palms to warm up. Proceed with the massage. These oil blends can be used with a hot stone massage or with any other massage treatment.

YIELD: 1 cup

USAGE: During a massage, rub the mixture into the skin. Rinse off when the massage is over.

YIELD: ½ to ¾ cup

Eucalyptus Body Rub

This creamy treatment invigorates as it moisturizes.

1 ripe banana

1 ripe avocado

4 drops eucalyptus essential oil

Peel the banana and avocado and mix with the eucalyptus oil in a blender on low speed.

Winter Spas

When it's winter:

❀ It's cold outside. It's warm inside.

❀ You decide you could live in your bathtub, if it wasn't for that little skin-wrinkling problem.

❀ Parties are everywhere, giving you excuses to buy floaty dresses and smokin' shoes.

❀ You love everyone, except those in line at the stores.

❀ You sleep a lot.

❀ You make a fort with blankets and chairs, and decide that skiing, sledding, and walking to your car are overrated.

❀ After the holidays, you waver between stir-crazy and just plain depressed.

❀ To counteract postholiday depression, you make far too many resolutions.

❀ You watch a lot of DVDs, perhaps in your fort.

❀ You sleep hard. When you wake up, you finish the juicy dream you were just having.

It's winter and you probably feel like a bear. You slumber, you just ate a meal that could carry you through to spring, your legs are a tad on the furry side, and you feel a bit uncoordinated. Winnie the Pooh often sighs, "Oh, bother," and that sums up your general outlook toward life right now. You hardly have enough energy to change the channel on your television . . . and you have a remote control!

Well, relax! The spas included in this section are the perfect antidote to the winter blahs. Without even getting off the couch, you and your guests can indulge in a reflexology massage. You can whip up some love potions to attract a hottie, even if you haven't shaved your legs in a month. Get pruney in a decadent bath. Winter is about soothing the spirit and the skin. With dark or snowy days outside, these spa parties are all about comfort and love.

It's critical to moisturize your face and skin, what

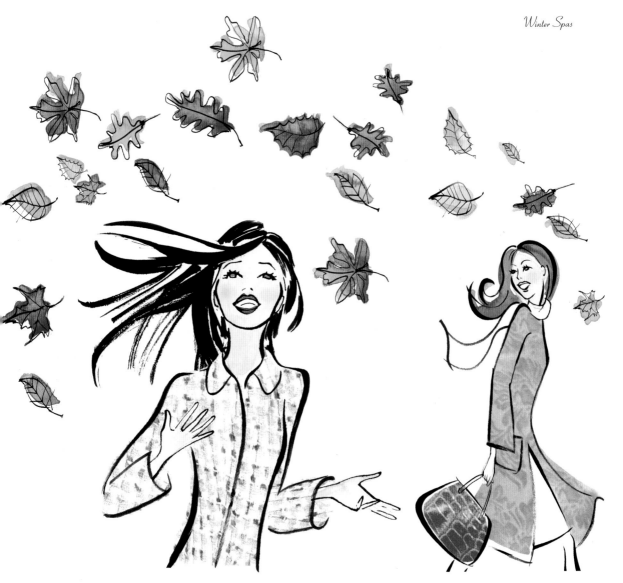

with winter's dry heat and cold, chapping weather. No matter the theme of your party, have thick body lotions and pitchers of water (or other tasty beverages) on hand. Ask your guests to bring along their favorite moisturizer as well. Hydration is key.

With so many special occasions dotting the winter months, there are plenty of opportunities for spa gatherings. Here are just a few reasons to celebrate winter in spa style:

CHRISTMAS: Color the party red and use peppermint as a key ingredient to rev up your guests for the holiday onslaught. Ask each guest to bring a small, wrapped spa-related treat. Put each in a basket and have guests choose a gift as they leave.

NEW YEAR'S DAY: Resolve to treat yourself and your friends better this year. Kick off your resolution with a New Year's Day party that does not include football games!

CHINESE NEW YEAR: Check online to see what animal is lording over the new year and toast to the monkey, snake, or rat with some oolong tea. Stretch with a few fluid tai chi movements and then pig out on takeout, complete with fortune cookies.

VALENTINE'S DAY: In a word, ugh. For this most heinous of days, take the guys out of the equation and schedule a spa party a month in advance. The pressure is off the guys and you and your friends will be guaranteed a night of primo TLC. Don't forget to shower them with chocolate, flowers, and pure love! Use the ideas in the Love Spa for inspiration.

AWARDS SEASON: For the Academy Awards (or the Golden Globes or Grammys), gather your friends together. Fill out ballots and treat the guest with the most winners to a reflexology massage and a toe ring with faux bling. Her feet will be camera-ready for her next red carpet appearance!

Game Day Spa

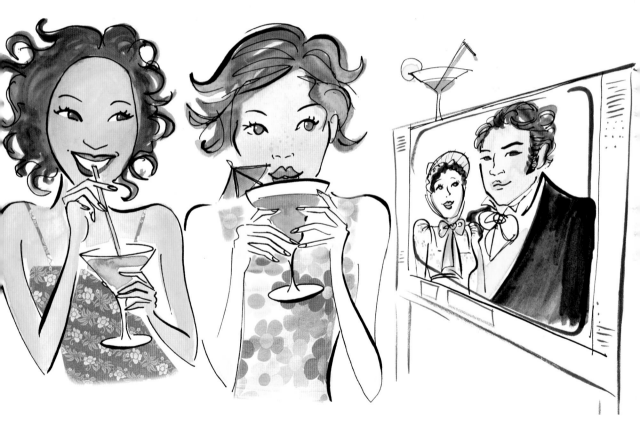

Outlet shopping and Internet dating may not be
Olympic sports yet, but they most certainly tire you
out as much as a football game. So while the boys are
watching the game, host a decidedly unsportsmanlike
party for your pals. With a *Sex and the City* or *Pride and
Prejudice* marathon in the background, or something else
totally girlie (think Go-Gos or Hilary Duff music), whip
up some pink cocktails and enjoy being a girl.

Gather your favorite sweet and savory snacks and
let your guests know that they get special dispensation
during the spa: they can gorge as freely as they like.
Cheese in any form is always a crowd pleaser. Stock your
freezer with more than a few pints of premium ice
cream. Pass around a platter of cupcakes or brownies.
Nothing is out of bounds!

As far as decor, throw in the towel on anything
vaguely sporty and opt instead for girlish touches. Create
a fort of femininity with bouquets of tea roses, lace-
trimmed tea towels, gingham tablecloths, and anything
that looks like it would be at home in Barbie's playhouse.

Give each friend a spray of pink flowers to take
home with her. Let them all enjoy being girls for as long
as possible.

Pizza Snacks

1 pound spicy Italian sausage

1 pound Velveeta cheese

3 tablespoons ketchup

Garlic powder and oregano to taste

1 loaf sliced party rye bread

Brown sausage in a skillet over medium heat. Drain and
return to burner. Turn down to low heat and melt in
cheese. Stir in ketchup and add garlic powder and
oregano to taste. Take off heat and allow to cool slightly.
Spread generously on bread slices. Bake at 400°F for
10 minutes or until top is browned.

YIELD: Serves 6 to 8

NOTE: The topping keeps for three weeks when refrigerated. You can also freeze the snacks and just pull out a few when you need a nibble.

Tea Tree Foot Scrub

This antiseptic scrub can also work wonders on elbows and rough hands. Just be careful not to use this magical mixture on any cuts.

    3 to 4 drops tea tree oil

    3 to 4 drops lavender essential oil

    3 to 4 drops rosemary essential oil

    1 teaspoon sweet almond oil

    1 cup coarse sea salt

Mix the oils together in a small bowl. Add sea salt and mix thoroughly with a clean metal spoon. Scoop into a jar or tub.

USAGE: This is a bit oily, so rub a handful over each foot in the shower or over a basin of warm water. Rinse off and pull on thick socks.

YIELD: One 8-ounce tub

NOTE: You could also do this after enjoying the Herbal Pine Foot Soak.

Spa Pedicure with Reflexology Massage

This deluxe treatment is rather time consuming for the hostess, so it might be a good idea to pair up guests and have them pamper each other. Who knows? They might just become sole-mates! (Sorry, I couldn't resist.)

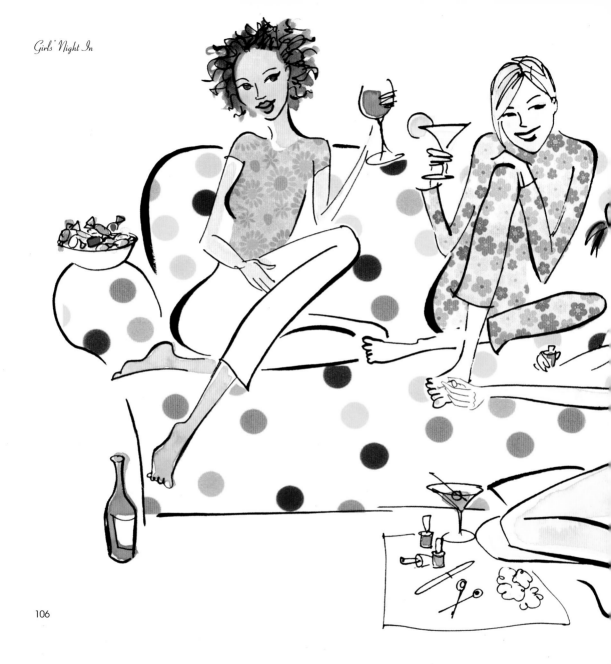

THE PEDICURE

Hand towel

Pumice stone or Tea Tree Foot Scrub

Orange stick

Emery board

Lotion or massage oil

Nail polish remover

Cotton balls

Facial tissue

1 bottle clear nail polish

1 bottle colored nail polish

Fill a basin with warm, soapy water and place it on a towel on the floor in front of your seated guest. Have her soak her feet for a few minutes. Rub her feet with a pumice stone or foot scrubber, focusing on the heels and calloused areas. Rinse her feet. One at a time, pat her feet dry with a hand towel and gently push cuticles back with an orange stick. File each nail with an emery board. The sturdiest shape is straight across and slightly rounded at the edges.

Massage lotion or oil into each foot and proceed with the Reflexology Massage. If you don't have time, lightly massage each foot with lotion until it's absorbed.

Dip a cotton ball into nail polish remover and wipe excess lotion from each toenail. Roll up a tissue and wind between each toe to separate. Apply a base coat to each nail and follow with two thin coats of color and a clear top coat. Wait a few minutes for the polish to dry and then clean up any errant polish by dipping an orange stick wrapped in cotton in nail polish remover. If necessary, fill a basin with cold water and dunk toes in it to quicken the drying process.

THE REFLEXOLOGY MASSAGE

The best part about this treatment? Long after you've rubbed your friends to spa nirvana, you can treat yourself to an amazing, effective foot massage whenever your dogs (or anything else) are barking. This reflexology massage comes from author and celebrity massage therapist Michelle Ebbin.

If you're not familiar with this wildly popular massage technique, here's the short version: Reflexology is the healing art of stimulating the feet to reduce stress and improve your physical well-being. Each foot contains more than 7,000 nerve endings, or reflexes, that correspond to every organ and system within your body. Simply pressing on those reflex points can elicit a response from the nervous system that helps to soothe and balance the entire body. Pretty cool, eh?

As you massage the feet, a weakness or imbalance in some area of the body may translate as tenderness in the corresponding reflex area on the foot. Pay attention to sensitive areas of your feet—they may require extra attention. There are several positions you can use when working on a guest.

THE COUCH: Sit face to face on opposite ends of a couch. Take one of your guest's feet in your hands and work on it. Place a pillow under her knees for extra support.

TIP: She can also massage your feet at the same time!

THE CHAIR: You might find it more comfortable to give treatments while sitting in a chair. If your guest is sitting on a couch or chair, or lying back on a massage table or bed, place your chair about 12 inches from the edge so you can comfortably take one foot in your hands without having to reach too far.

THE FLOOR: If you prefer to sit on the floor, have your guest either lean back against a wall or a couch, or lie down on her back. Place her feet on top of a firm pillow in front of you or in your lap. Remember, it's as important for you to be comfortable as it is for your partner to be relaxed.

ON TO THE MASSAGE ITSELF: Take some lotion or oil (see the massage oil blends) and warm it in your hands. Gently spread the lotion or oil over the top of the foot and the sole. Concentrate on the sole and work the lotion in so that there's only a light layer remaining. Apply precise pressure with your thumb all over the foot. Press firmly for about three seconds and then move to the next area. Press for a few seconds, then make small, circular motions. Stimulate all the reflex points on both feet to encourage the entire body to come back into balance. Refer to pages 110 and 111 for a guide to the pressure points and their corresponding body parts.

If your guest feels as if there are grains of sand under the skin or if an area is particularly tender, she may have some congestion in the corresponding part of her body. Give extra attention to this area.

TIP: During a massage, breathe deeply and slowly. You can also pick a color to think about as you inhale and exhale. To relax, think of lavender or deep blue. To revive, think of a spicy red or orange.

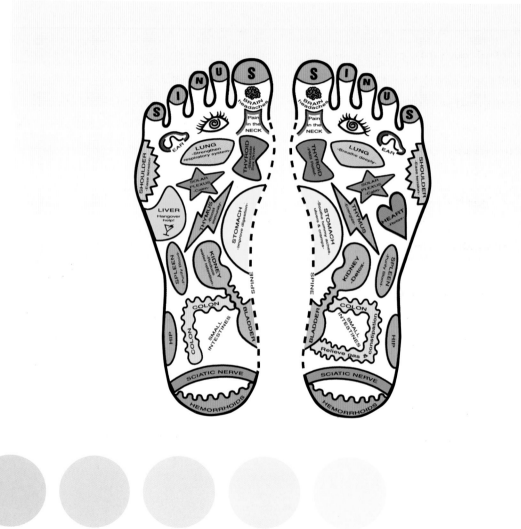

FEET: THE MIRROR OF YOUR BODY

BLADDER: reduce and ease bladder problems

BRAIN: stimulate sensory receptors, improve circulation, and relieve headaches

COLON: assist in the elimination of waste products, relieve gas and constipation

EARS: reduce pressure and open passageways

EYES: stimulate the optical nerves

HEART: improve blood circulation, open your heart

HEMORRHOIDS: relieve pain from varicose veins in the, ugh, rectum

HIP: relieve hip problems and pain

KIDNEYS: detoxify and prevent bloating, promote balanced elimination of water and waste

LIVER: detoxify blood and improve fat digestion; help for hangovers

LUNG: relax chest area, deepen breathing, and strengthen respiratory system

NECK: relax and loosen neck muscles

SCIATICA: relieve pain from the nerve that runs from the base of the heel up to the buttocks

SHOULDER: relax and ease shoulder tension

SINUS: help clear congested or clogged sinuses

SMALL INTESTINE: improve absorption of nutrients and improve peristaltic action

SOLAR PLEXUS: balance the nervous system and restore calm

SPINE: loosen your spine to improve circulation and nerve flow

SPLEEN: purify and balance blood deficiencies

STOMACH: improve digestion; soothe tummy aches, ulcers, and cramps; encourage muscular activity and the production of gastric juices

THYMUS: energize and boost immunity

THYROID: regulate metabolism and mineral levels; relieve PMS and stimulate your sex drive

Slumber Spa

Give the holidays and yourself a rest. Take a break from the hustle and bustle of holiday shopping, parties, and long work hours. Invite your friends over for a night of pampering, giggling, and gossiping, followed by a morning of yummy breakfast treats. Create a fort, or at least lay out lots of cushions and blankets for your guests to lounge around on.

But this won't be a completely authentic sleepover—there will be no mean-spirited hijinks! Slumber parties are a whole lot more than wicked games of Light as a Feather, Stiff as a Board. I bet more than one of you has put a sleeping girl's hand in warm water (to make her pee, silly!) or stuck her training bra in the freezer. The only things frozen at this party should be the margaritas. Instead, focus on a juicy game of Truth or Dare. I suspect there are a couple of secrets you've been dying to pry out of your friends. Now's your chance!

Pull on your favorite pair of pajamas (mine have bumblebees on them) and instruct your guests to do the same. Lingerie masquerading as sleepwear is strictly verboten. No one should have someone else's firm boobs or butt thrown in her face.

Fill the room with the sounds of your adolescence, be it Leif Garrett, the *Grease* soundtrack, the Bangles, or New Kids on the Block. Keep a camera on hand to record any old-school dance stylings that crop up. This party is a chance to own up to your cheesy music!

And cheesy movies. Rent a stack of classic teen comedies such as *Some Kind of Wonderful*, *Better Off Dead*, and *Dirty Dancing*. No one better put Baby in a corner tonight! Also throw in a recent movie you haven't had time to see (*What a Girl Wants* and *The Princess Diaries* are both pretty darn cute).

When it comes to food, make a fresh bowl of guacamole and set it out with blue corn chips. Set up a taco bar, complete with cheese, shredded lettuce, meat,

tomatoes, onion, soft
and hard taco shells, and
several types of salsa.
Wash everything down
with margaritas. For dessert,
set up a sundae bar with all the
fixings. (It wouldn't hurt to have a
bag or two of Doritos and Oreos on
hand for late-night cravings.)

A sleep mask, dream journal, a new
pillow or pillowcases, and a bottle of
Love's Baby Soft all make
super party favors.

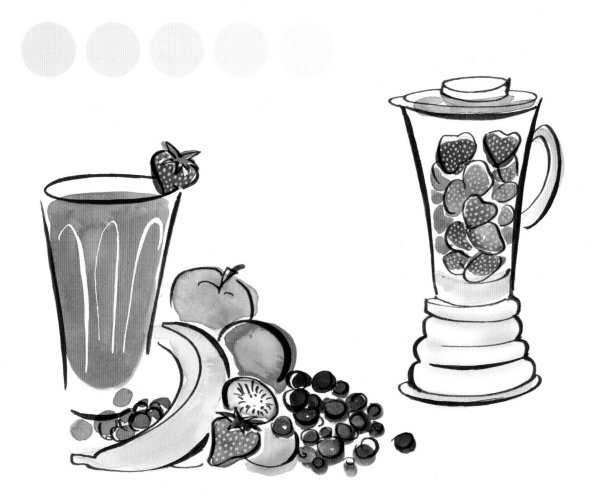

Mango Smoothie

This energizing breakfast treat is just what your guests need after your long night of beauty and debauchery.

¼ cup orange juice

1 cup nonfat vanilla yogurt

¼ mango, peeled and cut into small pieces

Several strawberries, sliced

Throw a few ice cubes and the orange juice into a blender and crush the ice. Add the yogurt and fruit and blend. Pour into a glass and enjoy!

YIELD: 1 smoothie

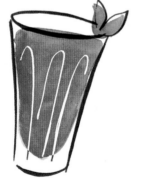

Creamsicle Bath

This dreamy creamy bath smells just like one of our favorite frozen treats from childhood. Send each guest into the bathroom for some quality alone time. Stock the bathroom with a pile of magazines, a stack of CDs, a portable stereo, and fluffy towels. Run a bath and pour a generous amount of this heavenly concoction under the tap. The milk will soften the skin and the sweet orange oil will prep your pals for sweet dreams.

½ cup powdered milk

1 tablespoon carrier oil, such as sweet almond or grapeseed oil

8 drops sweet orange essential oil

USAGE: Pour the powdered milk and carrier oil under the running tap as the bath is filling. Add the essential oil right before the bath is ready. Stir the water and climb in! Soak, pat dry, and finish with a light body lotion.

YIELD: 1 bath

Aromatic Facial Steams

This is an excellent way to prep the skin before a facial treatment. It opens the pores, allowing for better cleansing and moisturizing. Once a week, include this step as a special treat before applying a face mask or moisturizer.

DRY SKIN

3 cups water

½ teaspoon sweet orange essential oil

1 tablespoon sweet almond oil or jojoba oil

OILY SKIN

3 cups water

½ teaspoon clary sage essential oil

½ teaspoon peppermint essential oil

SENSITIVE OR MATURE SKIN

3 cups water

½ teaspoon rose essential oil

Boil water and pour into a plugged sink or large bowl. Add oils appropriate to your skin type.

USAGE: With a clean face and a towel over your head, lean over the sink so you are 10 to 12 inches from the steam mixture. Breathe deeply. Stay in this position for 5 to 10 minutes. Rinse your face with lukewarm water and follow up with your favorite moisturizer.

YIELD: 1 steam

Mango Hair Moisturizer with Cranial-Sacral Massage

While you could actually eat this, it will probably do more for your head than your palate. Remember to breathe in and enjoy the tropical fruit cocktail on your head.

1 vitamin E capsule

1 ripe banana

½ ripe mango

Puncture vitamin E capsule, peel fruit, and combine ingredients in a blender until thoroughly mixed.

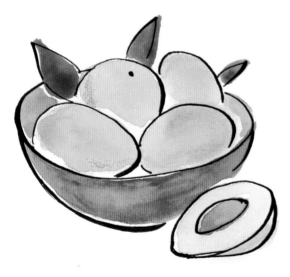

USAGE: Shampoo your guest's hair. While hair is still wet, comb the magic goo through. And so begins the head massage. Cranial-sacral massages manipulate the bones of the cranium and help regulate the rhythmic flow of cerebrospinal fluid.

Massage the back of the neck and head. This area is often very tight, and a good massage here can alleviate headaches and eye aches. Use thumbs and fingers to gently knead this area. Use a small, circular motion and work from the base of the neck up toward the head.

Move up toward the crown and sides of the head, using a basic thumb-walking technique: Apply precise pressure with your thumb (and fingertips). Press firmly for about three seconds and then move to the next area. Press for a few seconds, and then make small, circular motions. Move toward the ears and thumb-walk behind the ears but only gently tug on the earlobes themselves (ears can be very sensitive areas for many people). This tugging can actually help restore someone's equilibrium.

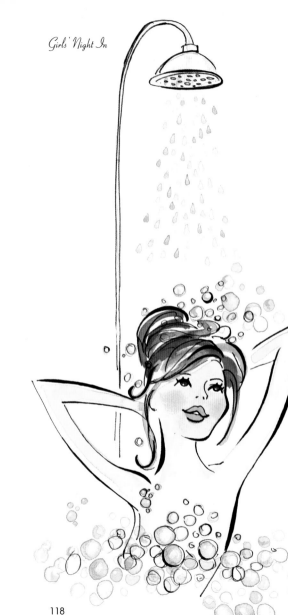

Now rub the temples slowly with your fingertips.

Moving to the face, with a flat hand stroke it with upward motions. Make sure to stroke the neck area as well. Rub your hands together quickly to create warmth from friction and complete the massage by gently sweeping your fingertips over your friend's closed eyelids. (You can do this to yourself whenever you want a sweet moment of calm.)

When done with the massage, cover hair with a shower cap for 20 minutes. Rinse with warm water and then wash as usual.

YIELD: 1 treatment

Love Spa

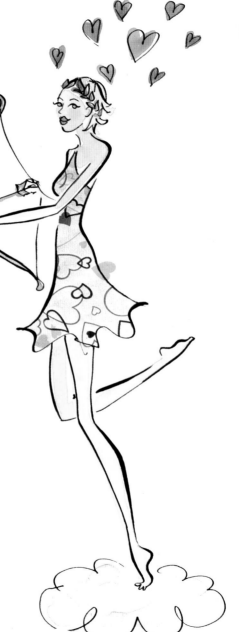

Celebrate with those who really adore you: your girlfriends! This is a perfect spa to host on the best and worst of holidays: Valentine's Day. Or host it on New Year's Eve and turn your back on the exhausting party circuit. Hand out sparkly tiaras or costume jewelry and count down to the new year at midnight. Ask your guests to make a wish for their love life in the new year.

You could have a burning ceremony during the party. Have your girlfriends go through magazines and rip out any words or images that they want to leave behind them or seek in the future. When each of you has a small pile, light each piece of paper and declare your intention as it goes up in smoke. Obviously, find a safe place to do this, be it an outdoor grill, a fireplace, or a stainless-steel sink.

If that's a bit too "out there" for you, just fill your house with red roses and votive candles. Sprinkle petals on the floor of your spa. Instruct guests to wear slinky pajamas or some other tactile clothing. Hand out journals so that guests can describe or sketch out their dreamboat.

Pass out champagne cocktails as you nibble on raw oysters, shrimp cocktail, or caviar-topped toasts. Follow up with chocolate-dipped strawberries or chocolate fondue. The rule of the day is decadence, especially when it comes to food!

As your guests leave, hand them a valentine, a rose, and a heart-shaped box of chocolates. You don't need a man to feel loved!

Champagne Cocktails

Just because it's a spa doesn't mean that you can't have some fizzy libations during your festivities.

6 ounces pink champagne

1 sugar cube

Dash of Angostura bitters

Twist of lemon

Hold a sugar cube over a bottle of Angostura bitters and invert the bottle so that some bitters soak into the sugar. Drop the cube into a champagne flute and fill the glass with champagne. Add a spiral of lemon twist.

YIELD: 1 cocktail

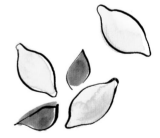

Here's another yummy pink concoction sure to please your friends.

1 tablespoon Chambord

6 ounces champagne

1 to 3 fresh raspberries

Pour the Chambord into a flute and fill the glass with champagne. Add a fresh raspberry or two.

YIELD: 1 cocktail

Perfect Pout Lip Balm

Forget about everyone else. Wearing this lip balm is guaranteed to make you fall in love with yourself. Not only does it smell like a peppermint patty, it will soften and protect your lips.

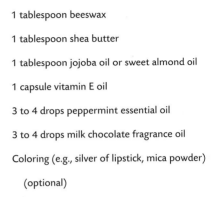

1 tablespoon beeswax

1 tablespoon shea butter

1 tablespoon jojoba oil or sweet almond oil

1 capsule vitamin E oil

3 to 4 drops peppermint essential oil

3 to 4 drops milk chocolate fragrance oil

Coloring (e.g., silver of lipstick, mica powder) (optional)

Melt beeswax and shea butter in a double boiler or in a glass measuring cup in a boiling pan of water. Add the jojoba/sweet almond oil. When all the ingredients are melted, remove from the heat and stir in the vitamin E oil, peppermint essential oil, milk chocolate fragrance oil, and coloring of your choice. Mix gently. Pour carefully into jars. Wait for the balm to cool before putting the lid on and moving the jars.

YIELD: Three ½-ounce jars

Customized Perfume Potions

Check out "Essential Oils: More than Just a Pretty Smell" on page 20 for information on various essential oils, their smells, and their properties.

Carrier oil

Various essential oils

Set up a table with various essential oils, a large bottle of carrier oil, a chart explaining the oils' properties, and one 1-ounce glass vial (available at health food and craft stores) for each guest. Fill each vial with 1 ounce of carrier oil. Each guest should add four drops of her favorite oil. If incorporating a second essential oil, add it one drop at a time until you are satisfied with the proportions. Close tightly, shake gently, and sprinkle a few drops on pulse points (neck, behind the ears, behind the knees, wrist, elbows). Each guest should breathe deeply and think about all the things she adores about herself.

A few winning combinations:

❀ Lavender and peppermint

❀ Juniper and sage

❀ Basil and mandarin

❀ Sandalwood and bergamot

❀ Ylang-ylang and patchouli

❀ Rose and jasmine are great by themselves

YIELD: 1 ounce per vial

NOTES: You can also pour a customized concoction into a small glass bowl to infuse your party with a delicious scent.

Do not blend more than three oils at a time. When working together, they can react and create effects that are different than those of the individual oils.

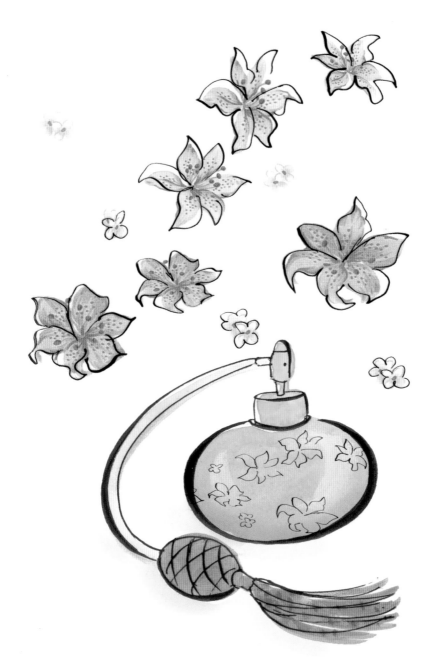

Resources

WEB SITES

www.aromaland.com Aromaland makes a wide range of essential oils and aromatherapy and spa products.

www.basicknead.com Celebrity massage therapist and author Michelle Ebbin runs this site, which offers information about reflexology and massage, and offers her massage videos, books, and patented reflexology and massage products.

www.beautyexclusive.com Check out these terrific spa treats if you want to forgo making your own lotions and potions.

www.fromnaturewithlove.com You can purchase ingredients such as essential and fragrance oils, shea butter, packaging, and even iridescent mica powders to tint your products. The site even features a library, so you can bone up on the properties and uses of various ingredients.

www.frontiercoop.com Features my favorite line of essential oils—Aura Cacia—as well as organic herbs, spices, teas, and foods. There are some good basic articles on aromatherapy if you want to learn more about the properties and benefits of various oils.

www.holistic.com This informative site can help you locate a practitioner in your area.

www.holisticonline.com This is one of several excellent Web sites if you want to explore any spa treatment in depth.

www.spafinder.com This online version of a leading spa magazine can help you locate a spa or guide you through various spa treatments.

BOOKS

Arvigo, Rosita. *Spiritual Bathing: Healing Rituals and Traditions from Around the World.* Berkeley: Celestial Arts, 2003.

Borgman, Peggy Wynne. *Four Seasons of Inner and Outer Beauty: Rituals and Recipes for Wellbeing Throughout the Year.* New York: Broadway, 2000. Spa professional Borgman presents lovely rituals to mark the changing seasons. Her goddess feast is particularly magical.

Kluck, Michelle. *Hands on Feet: The New System that Makes Reflexology a Snap.* Philadelphia: Running Press, 2001. This book comes with your very own pair of Reflexology Sox.

Kluck, Michelle. *The Little Book of Reflexology.* Philadelphia: Running Press, 2001. A pocket-sized book so you can massage on the go.

Lad, Vasant. *The Complete Book of Ayurvedic Home Remedies.* New York: Three Rivers Press, 1999. A great all-around introduction to Ayurveda.

Melody. *Love Is in the Earth: A Kaleidoscope of Crystals.* Earth Love Pub House, 1995. This is a comprehensive paperback that profiles every crystal, gem, and rock known to man. Look up a gemstone you love and be amazed at how much it reflects your personality or emotional state.

Tourles, Stephanie. *The Herbal Body Book.* Pownal, VT: Storey Publishing, 1994. Features a slew of easy home-spa recipes.

Acknowledgments

I cannot thank the following women enough for their invaluable contributions to this book. In researching this book and learning to make my own potions and do my own spa treatments at home, I am going to save a boatload of money. So ladies (and gentleman), I thank you and my burgeoning bank account thanks you!

Peggy Wynne Borgman, owner of Preston Wynne Day Spa and a school for spa management in Northern California, and the author of *Four Seasons of Inner and Outer Beauty*

Amy DiLuna, friend and in-the-know editor at the *New York Daily News*

Michelle Kluck Ebbin, massage therapist, author, and founder of Basic Knead (www.basicknead.com)

Babs Harrison, public relations diva and vice president at Sheila Donnelly and Associates

Kim Marshall, owner of the Marshall Plan, a communications company specializing in spas and resorts

Penny Ordway, founder of Eviama Day Spa in Philadelphia, Pennsylvania

Jacquelyn Overcash, founder of Get Fresh (www.getfresh.net)

Alison Rooney, best friend and all-around woman in the know

Stephanie Sakoff, founder/president of Lucky Chick (www.luckychick.com)

Kate Wingard, friend and editor at *Self* magazine

Janet Chase, Alexa Hokanson, and *Annika Jackson* at Mii Amo: A Destination Spa at Enchantment Resort in Sedona, Arizona

Kerry Colburn, Laurel Rivers, and *Brian Perrin,* publishing professionals who are always equipped with tasty recipes, luscious libations, and ideas for maximum indulgence

Index